ID0848900

# Carrying
# the
# Black
# Bag

# Carrying
## the
## Black
## Bag

*A Neurologist's Bedside Tales*

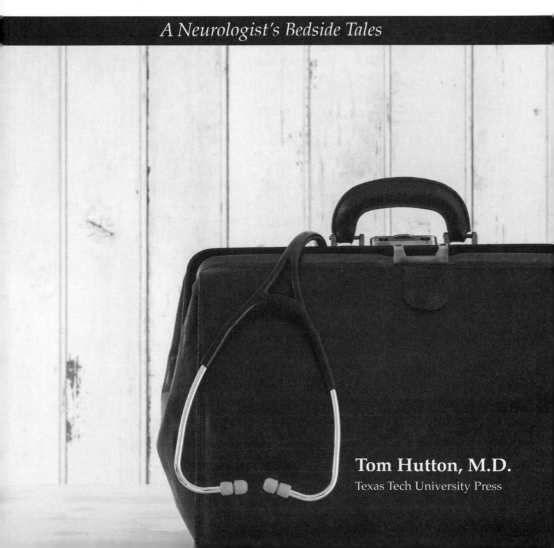

**Tom Hutton, M.D.**
Texas Tech University Press

This book is typeset in Palatino. The paper used in this book meets the minimum requirements of ANSI/NISO Z39.48-1992 (R1997). ∞

Designed by Kasey McBeath

Library of Congress Cataloging-in-Publication Data

Hutton, J. Thomas, author.
    Carrying the black bag : a neurologist's bedside tales / Tom Hutton.
        p. ; cm.
    Includes index.
    ISBN 978-0-89672-954-4 (hardback)
    I. Title.
    [DNLM: 1. Hutton, J. Thomas. 2. Neurology—Anecdotes. 3. Neurology—Autobiography. 4. Nervous System Diseases—Anecdotes. 5. Nervous System Diseases—Autobiography. WZ 100]
    RC339.5
    616.80092—dc23

                                                        2015028639

Printed in United States

15 16 17 18 19 20 21 22 23 / 9 8 7 6 5 4 3 2 1

Texas Tech University Press
Box 41037 | Lubbock, Texas 79409-1037 USA
800.832.4042 | ttup@ttu.edu | www.ttupress.org

# CONTENTS

Classical fables have archetypal figures—heroes, victims, martyrs, warriors. Neurological patients are all of these. . . . They are travelers to unimaginable lands—lands of which otherwise we should have no idea or conception.

Oliver Sacks, *The Man Who Mistook His Wife for a Hat: And Other Clinical Tales*

# ACKNOWLEDGMENTS

Many people have helped with this book, but my thanks especially go out to my patients, who entrusted their care to me and chose to share their amazing stories. From them I have learned invaluable lessons about life, death, and living with chronic illness.

I thank Alexander Romanovich Luria, my mentor in neuropsychology, who encouraged me to understand and write stories from the patients' perspectives. I owe much to my neurological mentor, A. B. Baker, chairman of the Department of Neurology at the University of Minnesota. I express my affection for Doctor William J. Powell, who showed me early on the excitement of medicine and how it benefits people's lives on a daily basis.

I wish to thank Don Fehr, who believed in this project from the beginning and helped make this book a reality. I am also grateful to my editor, Joanna Conrad, at Texas Tech University Press, and her associates, including Jada, Amanda, and Katherine, for making this a better book. What a wonderful experience to work with professionals who not only understand authors but also are consummate craftsmen and fun to work with. Making this book known has fallen into the highly capable hands of Maryglenn McCombs. I could not have possibly found someone more upbeat and capable.

Special and overdue thanks are due my wife, Trudy. Several times while deep in my writing, I lost any concept of time and left her stranded at a restaurant or a meeting. Her good humor and understanding of my absent-mindedness are acknowledged here and sincerely appreciated. She also, against her better judgment, became first reader on many of these chapters. Recognizing that an author should never, ever place a spouse in such a compromising position—I did it anyway, recognizing I could not possibly have a more exacting person for the job.

My heartfelt thanks go out to my family, including my children, Andy and Katie, who provided encouragement throughout the long writing process. I also thank the members of my extended family who sat through readings and fortified my early efforts. I acknowledge special gratitude to my parents, who made it possible for me to even consider a career in medicine.

I am grateful to friends who acted as readers, some of whom pored over earlier drafts. These include Janet, La Nelle, Nancy, Kent, Mara, Robert, Ottis, Vallie, Elizabeth, Tom, Allen, Susan, Stephen, Cecil, Betty, Nicky, Sarah, Noel, Patrick, Paul, and Ann. You all have been great.

My thanks go out to the doctors, nurses, and other health-care workers who appear in this book. Be assured, Susan, and at your insistence, I created the character of Vicki as thin and especially pretty. Nevertheless, your heart, your passion, and your full, head-on approach to life remain unequaled. To others who inspired characters within, I express my gratefulness. I also wish to recognize Rondine, Hillie, and Audrey for their efforts in establishing the Hennepin County General Hospital Museum and making available photos of the "Old General." Some other contributors may go unacknowledged due to oversight or special circumstances but are no less appreciated.

# Carrying
# the
# Black
# Bag

# PROLOGUE

Late in my senior year at Baylor College of Medicine, I received a much-anticipated message from the dean's office, prompting in me a geyser of exultation. The brief note said my black doctor's bag, embossed with my name followed by the treasured initials "MD," awaited my pickup. This notice carried momentous significance, as it showed that I was on the cusp of becoming a doctor. The black bag represented undeniable evidence that soon I would march among the ranks of physicians, including such legends as Hippocrates, Jonas Salk, and Albert Schweitzer.

Having passed through the winnowing sieve of college premed, I had gained admission to medical school. After I had learned a wealth of minutiae in anatomy, physiology, and biochemistry and survived rigorous clinical rotations that must surely have grown my adrenals to the size of cabbages, this leather icon assured me that finally a future in medicine lay just ahead.

On retrieving my black bag, I departed the heavily oaked Texas Medical Center in Houston and motored east on Old Spanish Trail. During the drive I was largely oblivious to the intense traffic, so intent was I on showing my wife, Trudy, my new black bag. While I had felt strangely uncomfortable showing too much emotion in front of my fellow medical students, I knew that with Trudy, and in the confines of our tiny apartment, we could fully celebrate this milepost.

As I drove home that day, a flood of emotions washed over me. These included the shock on my first day of medical school when I cranked up from the formalin-filled metal tank the staring, wrinkled human cadaver on which, and in which, I would work for the next year. My emotional shudder soon faded, but never to the extent of a few of my classmates, who managed even to eat meals while dissecting.

I also remembered the feelings provoked by my ob-gyn rotation when asked if I minded participating in and performing abortions. I believed this a matter between the patient and doctor, but I had qualms about my own involvement. For days ambivalence reigned. After deliberation, I declined to participate, harboring a sense that life, at any stage, was sacrosanct.

Behind me too was the heady exuberance of delivering babies, tying and severing their umbilical cords, and gazing with awe upon those crying bits of pink wonderment. Unquestionably that rotation was my happiest in medical school.

Also in the past was my thrill at sitting in the old, musty lecture hall at the National Hospital (Queen Square) in London. There at Queen Square beginning in 1859 the greats of neurology had lectured and established the underpinnings for the specialty. The masterful clinicians that I observed during a student clerkship in 1971 had impressed me with their ability to tease out symptoms and identify telltale physical findings. And all of this was done with a theatrical flourish worthy of the London stage.

Those expert practitioners of neurology seemed to elevate neurological diagnosis to an art form. Not only did I gain an intellectual thrill, but also I acquired an awareness of the huge importance of listening to patients and carefully examining them. This encounter in that ancient amphitheater was for me akin to watching a master magician pull a fluffy white rabbit from a top hat. Such clinical magic affirmed for me that neurology would one day become my medical specialty.

At stoplights on that muggy spring day in Houston, I glanced at my new shiny doctor's bag on the car seat next to me. Since the age of sixteen, medicine had defined the circumference of my life. One of my earliest medical memories was of our general practitioner, Doctor William J. Powell, making house calls on the "under the weather" Hutton children. He carried with him his enormous black medical bag, from which he would extract exam instruments and healing medicines. His kind temperament, boundless sense of humor, endless patience, and vast knowledge planted the seed in me to become a doctor.

One of my later meetings with Doctor Powell, I recall less clearly. At age fifteen during a pregame baseball warm-up, I raced across the outfield attempting to snag a long fly ball. I later learned that I smacked headfirst into a light pole. This had created a sickeningly loud thud that hushed the yammering crowd.

My next memory is fuzzy but consists of hearing the wail of a siren as the ambulance raced across town to Doctor Powell's clinic. I vaguely recall Doctor Powell shining a bright flashlight in my eyes and scraping the soles of my feet. At the time I did not understand why he chose to do such odd things. Nevertheless, during the gradual process of regaining consciousness and in between episodes of retching, I was aware of the embracing warmth of his good humor.

On that spring day while driving to our apartment on the Gulf Freeway, I could not have known the excitement that lay ahead during my internship at Hennepin County General and my neurology residency at the University of Minnesota. I had come to realize by then our brains were potentially capable of creating wonderful literature, finding cures for devastating diseases, or altering the course of world history. Other organ systems, it seemed to me, served less august functions, such as the kidney making urine, the liver metabolizing food, and the heart pumping blood. The brain struck me as the ultimate organ for thought and creativity and invited a more intimate, stimulating, and personal doctor-patient relationship.

I would become evermore hostage to the brain's siren enticement and its engendering of peculiarities in the face of disease. I had already witnessed how a deficiency of a brain chemical transmitter, dopamine, could result in a patient who was stooped, unable to walk, tremulous, stiff, and slow moving. I had marveled at the dramatic reanimation that occurred when the man with Parkinson's disease received L-dopa. After the first few days of treatment, as if by a miracle, he stood up, walked, and moved much more fluidly.

My hand stole across the seat and stroked the leather bag. I felt the coolness of the buckle and the irregular indentations in the leather. I lifted and dropped the handle, prompting a subtle thumping sound as it struck the side of the empty bag. I, like the bag, was largely empty of what it would take to become a competent neurologist.

From observing patients and from reading, I had marveled at how an abnormal electric discharge in the brain could create strange smells, vivid memories, arrests in speech, strange sensations, and unwanted muscle contractions. Even more intriguing I found were the mystical experiences described in people with epileptic seizures and by patients at the time of neurosurgery with direct electrical stimulation to their brains.

One remarkable description stuck in my memory. Fyodor Dostoyevsky had recounted that his seizure aura created moments of utter bliss, the pleasure of which was so intense that he would have traded the remainder of his life for a mere prolongation of the ecstatic moment. Following this the poor man would fall unconscious during a generalized convulsive seizure that was followed by days of the deepest, darkest despondency.

I had no way to know in 1969 that my future would include studying with Academician A. R. Luria at the University of Moscow. Luria, who would mentor me in neuropsychology, and Doctor A. B. Baker at the University of Minnesota, who would train me in neurology, became the major influencers of my professional life. It was from Luria, the greatest living Soviet neuroscientist of his day, that I learned not only the facts of neuropsychology but also the importance of viewing patients' stories from their unique perspectives. He had resurrected this age-old approach to medical storytelling largely from nineteenth-century traditions, and he had penned such moving psychodramas as *The Mind of a Mnemonist* and *The Man with a Shattered World*.

One afternoon during the late 1980s, I enjoyed a memorable several-hours-long telephone conversation with the American neurologist and author Oliver Sacks, who had continued the Lurian writing tradition. The purpose of my telephone call had been to enlist Sacks as a commencement speaker for the Texas Tech School of Medicine. My invitation was quickly declined, as he, just then, was in the midst of shooting the film *Awakening*. He shared with me that the movie, based on his book of the same name, would star Robert De Niro and Robin Williams. Our wide-ranging conversation included whether or not De Niro could really be coached into acting as though he suffered from parkinsonism (he could very nicely, as it turned out).

What irony that Robin Williams, who played the role of treating physician for De Niro's character, would later develop Parkinson's disease. Like so many other sufferers of this disorder, the prelude to Williams's movement disorder was depression. Doubly ironic was that this talented comedian, who had caused great laughter and joy for so many, suffered from such deep despair that he took his own life.

During our telephone conversation, Sacks also shared his persistent longings to have spent time with the, by then, deceased Luria. He questioned me extensively in his good-humored, broad British accent about my year in Moscow with Luria and repeatedly shared his personal debt to Luria.

The epigraph quotation earlier in this book comes from Oliver Sacks's preface to his book *The Man Who Mistook His Wife for a Hat*. In Sacks's inimitable way, he describes neurological patients like archetypal and heroic figures, depicting widely fanciful lands, ideas, and conceptions. I love his metaphorical description, as it aptly describes the lives of many neurological patients.

As I hurried home that day in Houston with my new black bag, I had no inkling of the exhilaration that would come from caring for and learning from my future patients. The chapters that follow continue the Lurian tradition of telling stories from their perspective. My stories are real and describe people afflicted by illnesses as told from my forty years as a practicing physician. My accounts describe remarkable people who faced life-threatening or life-altering illnesses such as Parkinson's disease, stroke, seizure disorders, Alzheimer's disease, Reye's syndrome, and other serious or not so serious maladies. Many of these people responded in unique and inspiring ways that enlarge our consideration of the human condition.

The medical anecdotes that follow will also provide insights into faith, love, hope, and most of all, courage. Love has the utmost importance in the lives of ill people. Having witnessed easy deaths and deaths of those who struggled to the end, I remain convinced that those capable of expressing love had the easier deaths.

An elderly, life-weary couple you will meet later in the book impressed on me the importance that love has in our lives. They were from the fringe of society, devoid of wealth or attractiveness, but managed to maintain their bond to the very end—a union that gave their shared lives both meaning and sustenance.

I write of the importance of hope for patients and their caregivers. Hope supports the patient and family, empowers caregivers, and sometimes leads to unexpectedly merciful outcomes. Hope fuels the will to live and strengthens the efforts of caregivers. To a degree the doctor-patient relationship also pivots around such hope—hope that sustains the patient and hope tempered by the doctor's scientific knowledge.

Over my career I found observing people with neurological disorders much like watching a person at a poker table pushing all his chips into the middle for a final, "all in" bet. Unfortunately, people with serious brain diseases usually lose, but sometimes and against seemingly insurmountable odds, they win. Lacking a miracle cure, however, I found most patients desired a means for preserving their dignity and reducing the hurtful impact on their loved ones.

I recall a sandy-haired, middle-age businessman dying from ALS (amyotrophic lateral sclerosis, or Lou Gehrig's disease). He, like most other people with this terrible condition for whom I cared, held a degree of hope that a cure would arrive in time, but also shared that he wanted to avoid futile, life-prolonging, terminal care. He wanted to spare his family the expense and ordeal of terminal respirator care and daily tube feedings. I have always been struck by the unselfishness and courage some patients muster while facing the specter of their own deaths, eschewing futile, but life-prolonging medical care.

In my neurology practice, unfortunately I found thorny life-and-death issues all too prevalent. However, in addition to rich pathos and poignancy, some patients also exhibited humor—an odd sort of humor that made light of symptoms, foibles, and failing abilities and demonstrated a healthy acceptance and a secure emotional balance. One brassy Texas homemaker suffering from severe, rhythmic hand tremor from Parkinson's disease took power over it by boasting of her tremor's benefit for shaking martinis and for providing excellent sexual foreplay.

The other half of the doctor-patient relationship is, of course, the doctor. Like patients, doctors and nurses also use humor in treating persons with grave illnesses, and at times we resort to bizarre escapades to lighten a downcast mood. Such was the case when a dripping, motorcycle-riding intern colleague arrived at the pediatric ward still covered by his rain gear, a black trash bag with cutouts for eyeholes. A lighthearted nurse approached him with a concerned patient's family in tow. The nurse stepped aside as she pointed to the wet, dripping trash bag and portentously announced, "And here's your eminent doctor!"

Doctors and nurses are, after all, human beings with the same feelings and vulnerabilities as anyone else, although often appearing as if encased by impermeable veneers. What creates these emotional barriers and why they exist may in part be defensive in nature, allowing physicians to function with greater objectivity. Nevertheless, emotional standoffishness, in my opinion, separates those perceived as cold or uncaring from those with stellar bedside manners.

Little has been written about how physicians deal with the immense responsibility of having patients' well-being entrusted to their care. A patient's trust is a precious and delicate commodity. I found it like holding a baby bird in my hand. It had to be done gently and with a loving nature. Little also has been written about the scientific methods that direct doctors' work. Physicians use deductive reasoning to diagnose. The effort involves searching the patient's story for nuanced clues and drawing increasingly stronger conclusions as mounting history, physical exam, imaging, and laboratory evidence allows.

In 1974, at the beginning of my fellowship on the US-USSR Health Exchange Program to the University of Moscow, I asked Professor Luria what he considered to be good preparation for becoming a neuropsychologist and neurologist. The eminent clinician surprised me by answering that reading mysteries was a fine background. He revealed that identifying and cobbling together clues was really no different for making neurological diagnoses than it was for solving crimes. Sherlock Holmes and Hercule Poirot, I suppose, would have made fine neurologists.

Modern health care can also have its drawbacks. How many of us lately have experienced our physician spending more time typing on his laptop and staring at his computer screen than making eye contact with us or examining us? Worryingly, more physician effort may go into checking all the necessary boxes to justify the complexity level for a specific billing code than in determining clues to establish a useful medical record. Don't get me wrong; I believe electronic medical records (EMR) is a wonderful technology. However, it is better suited for billing and case aggregation for research purposes than it is for building a medical record for patient care and maximizing the doctor-patient relationship.

I think the practice of medicine is, and always will be, the human-to-human transfer of information and the rendering of care. The art of medicine, which is at the heart of the discipline, requires good listening and careful communication. It will continue to be as important in the future as will the evolving technological advances.

Scattered databases for nurses and doctors in the EMR without proper communication among the medical team will inevitably lead to medical errors. As I write this, such errors are being found to underlie the Ebola transmission from the patient from Liberia to two nurses in Dallas. Careful person-to-person instruction within the health-care team on the proper use of protective gear and continued use of person-to-person, end-of-shift conferences might have prevented the spread of this terrible virus.

Effective communication, as I shared at the midnight meal described in a later chapter, hopefully provides more than a nostalgic story of what occurred in the middle of the night among tired interns and residents. If the midnight meal is no longer feasible, then other means will be needed to provide opportunities for an effective exchange of ideas among health-care workers. Effective communication will become the driver of improved patient safety and quality of care.

Real events and patients inspired every story in this volume. The time frames may have been compressed, settings altered, names changed, and at times characters merged due to privacy concerns. I also invented a few minor characters to benefit the storytelling. While the identities and circumstances of patients have been altered to preserve privacy, all the stories are emotionally true.

As I examine the decades encompassed by this book and during which I carried a black bag, I also recognize a change in myself. The initial high anxiety accompanying my first intern rotation in the neonatal intensive care unit contrasts my more confident approach decades later. It was a great but, at times, tumultuous ride. The symphony of physician experiences, some better than others, season and mature all of us.

As if naked, I stand before the reader, as an evolving physician. Initially young, naïve, and ambitious, I moved through a period of intense knowledge acquisition and finally experienced a period in which I became a more insightful healer. Somewhere in the scaffolding of my becoming a physician, the hard science learned became overlaid with awe for the indefatigable human spirit. While requiring time and some work on my part, much of it came from daily contact with my patients.

Harkening back to that hot and muggy spring day in 1972, Trudy and I celebrated my first medical black bag by partaking of the Friday night all-you-can-eat special at the nearby Howard Johnson's. Over the next several months I carefully gathered and placed into the black bag a stethoscope, otoscope, ophthalmoscope, tourniquets, materials for sensory testing including tufts of cotton, tuning forks, and a special hat pin found only in an out-of-the-way London hat shop, tongue blades, adhesive and paper tape, and a reflex hammer. At night the bag with its special contents occupied a corner of my study desk, ready at a moment's notice to depart for the hospital.

To paraphrase Oliver Sacks, the medical bag would soon accompany me on a long journey that would take us to strange lands of which otherwise I would have never gained any conception or idea.

Please join me now on this journey and meet those people whose lives prompted my professional sojourn. Learn about their reservoirs of courage and perseverance, and about their struggles to achieve balance for their disrupted lives. In the final analysis, these stories offer a voice for people who no longer can speak for themselves.

Step closely, as often they speak with low and muffled voices but voices that nonetheless ring loudly with humanity, love, hope, and most of all, courage.

*Chapter 1*
# OF MIDDLE LINEBACKERS
# AND MEDICINE

*Of a good beginning cometh a good end.*

—John Heywood

In part my choice of vocation should be credited to a beefy
middle linebacker who played for the Richardson (Texas) High
School football team. Without his assist, I would likely have become the attorney my parents had hoped. I never did send the
brawny backer a thank-you card, because even after fifty years,
the memory remains too painful.

I recall the story like this. In August of 1962, the Richardson
High football team began two-a-day summer practices in the
August heat. I was at the time a light-in-the-britches 145-pound
wannabe running back with ambition far outstripping my talent. To identify players with the most aggressive tendencies, the
coaches organized a one-on-one tackling drill that seemed to
me akin to a human demolition derby. Two players hemmed
in by blocking dummies faced off from five yards apart. On the
coach's signal, the ball carrier plowed ahead while the other
player attempted to tackle him. I recall that with particularly
violent collisions, the coaches would whoop it up like wild ban-
shees.

Eventually I worked my way to the front of the line. When I
gazed across the line, my eyes must have enlarged to the size of
truck tires when I spotted the bruiser. Before me hulked Butch,

compressing the football in his hands as if it were a beach ball. He sneered before tucking the ball away in the crook of his elbow. This star senior middle linebacker, destined to become all-district, packed 230 pounds of muscle on his five-foot eleven-inch frame. He looked to me like an enormous human bowling ball without finger holes.

The coach ordered me down into a three-point stance. I felt no escape but was hesitant to place my hand on the ground. But what else could I do before such weighty authority and peer pressure? Out of the corner of my eye, I viewed a sinister leer on the face of the head coach. The linebacker leaned forward and gave a guttural snarl, reminding me of a lion's anticipatory, satisfied growl prior to ripping into his prey. I took a resigned breath and after a few interminable seconds the coach yelled, "Hut."

What happened next was likely a testament to blind luck. I charged ahead, possessing a faster start than did the stocky, muscled-up one. It simply took him time to accelerate that much mass. Before he could take more than a step or two, I struck him in the legs like a slender arrow striking the treads of a Sherman tank. I somehow managed to entangle my reedlike self between his stumplike, churning legs. The stocky one's forward progress slowed, and soon I sensed him begin to totter. He lost his balance, pitched forward, and crashed to the turf like a mighty fallen oak.

From the crowd of players and coaches rose a collective gasp of amazement. The scrawny sophomore had actually tackled the team's Goliath. Any affirmation was lost on me, as all I felt was a terrific pain from a newly acquired, nonanatomical positioning of my left thumb. My fledgling career on the varsity football team had just been crushed, as surely as had my thumb.

An hour later, I was riding with my mother in her 1959 boatlike Buick Le Sabre that possessed tailfins the size of DC-3 wings.

"Where're you taking me?" I grumped while gingerly holding my aching hand.

"To Doctor Powell's. He's a great doctor and he'll fix you up."

"I know I could've made the team. All those wind sprints and for what?"

"Now, son, keep in mind when one door closes, another always opens." That was vintage Mom—the eternal optimist.

Just then I was not remembering any doors opening, just all those push-ups and sit-ups. I assumed her reference to an opening door was that of Doctor Powell's medical clinic located just off Main Street in Richardson, Texas. When it had swung open for me months before, I had been unconscious.

As a ninth-grade baseball player, I had been ambulanced to Doctor Powell's office after pursuing a fly ball headlong into an unforgiving light pole. My buddies later teased me, claiming irredeemable stupidity for having steamed full bore into a post. I viewed it merely as my great ability to focus on the job at hand.

Doctor Powell, a trained surgeon who also practiced general medicine, had served as our family doctor since our arrival in Texas in 1957. The bespectacled, rumpled physician with an ever-present bow tie and expensive dress shoes bore an eccentric appearance in Texas where string ties and boots were considered high fashion. I could not have known at the time that I would spend much of the following month within the confines of his clinic.

The holdup resulted from a distinct difficulty in setting my mangled thumb. The stubborn fragments failed to line up like good little soldiers, instead choosing to scatter like leaves before a gusty Texas wind.

"Now, Tom, just don't like the alignment of these bone chips," he would say. "Will nudge the fragments a little bit more." Doctor Powell would make such comments while scrutinizing X-ray films on the view box. His idea of "nudging a bit" felt as if he were tying my thumb bones into square knots.

Doctor Powell was a painstaking perfectionist. Over the course of four weeks, he repeatedly set, then rebroke, and again set the aching bones of my thumb. The exposing and developing of X-rays and the casting and recasting of my fracture required many long and uncomfortable days within his clinic.

One afternoon, Doctor Powell stuck his head into the waiting room where I sat. "Tom, bet you've read those old magazines by now and are getting a might bored?"

"Well, I would like something else to do."

"Interested in seeing patients with me?" And that is how it all began. By and large, the patients accepted my presence without question. I should mention that privacy concerns were much less appreciated in those days.

I followed Doctor Powell down the hallway to his break room where I claimed a folding chair, but I would pop up anytime he headed toward an exam room. Between patient visits, while breathing in the antiseptic aroma of the clinic, I pestered Doctor Powell and Nurse Margaret with a litany of teenage questions.

"How does the autoclave work?"

"What's the trick to drawing blood?"

"What time do you start your hospital rounds?

"Doesn't the sight of blood make you queasy?"

"Aren't you afraid of catching something?"

"How can you tell on X-ray if the bones are mending?"

Nurse Margaret, the antithesis in personality to Doctor Powell's casualness, proved prompt, well organized, and thoroughly starched. Her Germanic organizational skills kept the clinic humming with a minimum of disruptions. She fortunately possessed a motherly forbearance of youthful questioners.

Between his patients, Doctor Powell continued to place pressure on my recalcitrant, maverick bone fragments. As I recall, that month I held hands with Doctor Powell so much that my girlfriend got jealous. But little did I know that keeping close to Doctor Powell would prove the engine for my ultimate career choice.

The days shadowing Doctor Powell allowed me to gain insight into the day-to-day workings of a medical practice. I observed him proceeding at his own deliberate pace, chatting up patients, planning investigations, passing out prescriptions, and scheduling surgeries. When decisions needed to be made, Doctor Powell made them without delay or pleadings to higher powers. It was clear, he treasured the independence of his solo practice.

It was also obvious that Doctor Powell enjoyed the respect and affection of his patients. My summer's sojourn in the clinic allowed me to meet many of his patients, but three encounters were especially memorable.

Wendell Newberry was an elderly farmer and part-time shade tree mechanic. In addition to his unsolicited complaints about the sorry state of the world with its sordid inhabitants, he also possessed numerous bodily concerns. After explaining the presence of the fresh-faced sixteen-year-old with the short-arm, wet-plaster cast, Doctor Powell inquired about Mr. Newberry's medical concern.

"Can't pee worth a diddly damn," Wendell blurted, his jaw jutting out pugnaciously. "Used to pee a damned rope, could drill a red ant from six feet. Now dribble on my own damned shoes. Ain't fun walking around in soggy shoes neither!"

"Have you any difficulty getting your stream started or having it cut off unexpectedly?"

"Doc, at my age damn near everything's unexpected, like waking up in the morning. But now you mention it, wait awhile worshipping at the porcelain throne—mind you, ain't standing holding my manhood to pass the time of day." He said all this with a gruff tone.

"Any burning when you pass your urine," asked Doctor Powell.

"Nah, just a feeling of bona fide accomplishment," said Wendell, smiling at his witticism, as he rubbed his hand across his three-day stubble.

"How's the sexual performance?" asked Doctor Powell.

"Done up and gone. Would be a miracle; heavens would part and choirs of angels would sing hosannas," retorted Wendell. I could not help but turn my head away and chuckle quietly.

Later I was still sniggering in the break room when Doctor

Powell explained the possibilities for Mr. Newberry's prostate symptoms. He explained this while writing down various tests for Nurse Margaret to order. I remember feeling impressed that the doctor had sifted through Wendell Newberry's heaps of verbiage to discover telling diagnostic clues. I could not have been more impressed had I just met the governor.

About a week later a completely different caliber of patient appeared. Eddie Mae Jones was only fifty-five but looked on the high side of seventy. She wore her dull gray hair pulled back in a tight bun and dressed in loose-fitting clothing in brown hues. Mrs. Jones appeared timid and spoke so softly that I had to take a step closer to hear her. She avoided eye contact with both Doctor Powell and me. I wanted to like this doughty grandmother type, but she had a whiney, nasal voice that proved as off-putting as rap music at a wedding.

"Well, Eddie Mae, how have you been doing these last few weeks?" Doctor Powell began. The thickness of her chart indicated she was paying more than her fair share of the clinic's overhead.

"Oh, Doctor Powell, those stomach pills were wonderful. Am feeling so much better." While her words sounded positive, her inflection was as flat as a table.

"Well, what brings you to the clinic today?"

"Doctor Powell, I'm having awful headaches all the time." The tone of her voice, her downcast eyes, and her gloomy countenance were by then making me as sad as when my blind, old dog had wandered off and gotten lost. Eddie Mae had a way of saying things that implied abject powerlessness and victimization.

"I see. Is the pain still in the front of your head and in your neck, Eddie Mae?"

"Yes, something squeezing my head—like a vice crimping down hard." She made a squeezing gesture with her hands.

Doctor Powell stood up and walked behind the gray metal chair in which she slumped. He began to palpate and rub muscles in Eddie Mae's neck. He guided her head from side to side, then down and up.

"Neck feels tense, Eddie Mae. Now what's going on with you?" Before she responded, he went on to ask, "By the way, how's that husband of yours these days?"

"Oh, Bill's okay. Has his own ways, you know."

"Well, Eddie Mae, is Bill angry and yelling at you like a few months back?"

She was slow to respond, as if measuring her words.

"Well, I suppose. I bring a lot of it on, though. Gets plumb irritated with me, he does."

"Eddie Mae, you strike me as looking sad. Am I right? You feeling down in the dumps?"

Another brief pause occurred before Eddie Mae responded in her low-pitched and hesitant way.

"Well, guess my spirits are kinda low. Just don't have any energy."

It was then that I witnessed a never-to-be-forgotten act. Doctor Powell walked around and sat down at eye level with Eddie Mae, staring intently and kindly at her. He ignored Nurse Margaret's rattling of the doorknob, her signal it was time to move along. He began to carry out a desultory conversation that at first seemed aimless. Eventually he reached forward and grasped Eddie Mae's unadorned, chapped, reddened hands. He caught her gaze and in a resonant, emotion-filled, and quaking voice said, "Eddie Mae, you're a good person. And ah, ah, I like you. I'm glad to have, have you as, as, *as a friend.*"

Eddie Mae's face blossomed into a beaming, warm expression. For the first time, she raised her eyes and fixed them on Doctor Powell's smiling countenance. I noticed her shoulders lower and her posture improve.

Later in the break room I commented on Eddie Mae's remarkable physical and emotional reaction to his powerful words.

"Well, Tom, no matter what field of medicine a doctor chooses, he will see depressed patients. Folks like Eddie Mae get loaded up with sacks of medicines and unnecessary surgeries. By the way, those wonder pills, helped her stomach so much? Placebos, inactive sugar pills. Sometimes doctors must address emotional needs, as depression gives rise to all kinds of strange symptoms. The treatment, as with Eddie Mae, may be as simple as sharing a personal conversation—saying simply that you like them. An antidepressant medicine helps but I'll wait for now on that. Loneliness is common these days and can best be addressed by human contact and friendship. Not as exciting as dealing with a runaway, blood-spurting artery, but a doctor can help a bunch by understanding the real needs of folks. I like to think of this approach as the doctor's personality becoming like a medicine. Tom, don't ever underestimate the impact of a caring voice and a kind attitude on a depressed person."

Even at the age of sixteen, I knew his words were profound. "I noticed your voice began to quiver," I said.

"Glad you noticed," Doctor Powell said. "Think it's a nice touch."

I was stunned. Not only had I seen a masterful clinician at work, but I may have witnessed a consummate actor as well. Eddie Mae's visit became a lesson never to be forgotten. Later in my professional life, Doctor Powell's advice often proved helpful, indeed some of the best counsel I ever gained from a skilled clinician.

Ten days later, before entering another exam room, Doctor Powell shared with me that he had begun performing cosmetic surgery. In the early sixties it was just entering upon the medical scene. Doctor Powell had gained additional training and was trying his hand at this new surgical technique. Nannette Martin, the next patient, represented one of his early efforts.

As compared to Eddie Mae, Nannette possessed a drastically different personality and appearance. This brassy mid-thirties woman had returned to the clinic following surgery a week before. She had long, raven hair, mischievous brown eyes, sparkly jewelry with huge golden hoops in her ears, and heavily accented makeup. Nannette wore a loose, low-cut, flowered white blouse and short, candy-apple-red leather skirt. Her seductive scent would have weakened the knees of any man. She was a head turner—very much different from the high school girls I knew.

"Nannette, how're you doing?"

"A little sore but otherwise great. Had wonderful comments and, wow, have I gotten some looks." She purred out these words with a coy smile on her face. "Well, I just wiggle my hips and stare right back."

"No suture breakdowns or bleeding?" Doctor Powell asked.

"Nah. Now, Doctor Powell, who's this young stallion with you?" she said flirtatiously, lasering her gaze squarely on me. The way she was looking at me made me feel unsettled, causing me to take a small step backward.

"This is Tom. He's seeing patients with me. Tom, Nannette just underwent mammoplasties."

"Mammo-whats?" I said.

"Breast augmentation. She was flat-chested, self-confidence affected. Having self-esteem issues she was. We decided to fix all that with an operation."

I noticed Nannette bore a proud look on her face, as if she had just won the grand prize for her preserves at the Texas State Fair. If she had indeed previously been shy, the surgery had transformed her as much as Professor Henry Higgins had Eliza Doolittle.

"Nannette, now let's get a look at my handiwork." With no more to-do than if she were flipping back her silky hair, she reached down and whipped up her blouse and arched her back to reveal swollen, oversized breasts. Her sudden flinging upward of her blouse had surprised me.

"Aren't they marvelous?" Nannette said with a huge smile on her face.

I stepped closer to inspect. At that proximity her strong perfume became more overwhelming. I felt light-headed and thought I might faint. My gaze attached to the two massive globes. I felt my face flushing. I wondered if my facial expression revealed whether I was inspecting Doctor Powell's handiwork or ogling her breasts. I was torn between searching for surgical evidence of Nannette's breast augmentation and mentally counting Herbies—an apocryphal measure of female breast size springing from the hormonally tortured minds of adolescent males and hypothetically calculated in cubic mouthfuls.

"Well, my young Tom, whaddaya think? You think these babies will get a guy's attention?" Nannette asked this in a seductive voice that momentarily dislodged my transfixed gaze from her breasts to her prideful face.

I was completely unaccustomed to having women throw up their blouses and show me their breasts, much less ask me for my approval. Words would simply not come from my suddenly muted mouth.

Around the circumference of her discolored orbs snaked precise blue suture lines. Her breasts and adjacent skin showed extensive swelling and bruising, explaining her lack of a bra. Her pink nipples on exposure to the cool exam room puckered up like tiny rosebuds. Nannette's face suggested she felt competitive with the likes of Marilyn Monroe and Brigitte Bardot.

"Well, Tom, how do you like my work?" asked Doctor Powell proudly, reminding me of an artist standing before his masterpiece.

With hindsight of fifty years, I wish I had possessed the presence of mind to compare Nannette's ample bosom to the beauty of a Gauguin painting or a Michelangelo sculpture, or at the very least have claimed her breasts were beautiful and the surgery impressive. I recall instead mumbling something like, "Wow, do they hurt?"

From each of these encounters I learned valuable lessons. From the truculent Wendell Newberry, whose mind appeared devoid of temperate zones, I witnessed the thrill of discovery in observing Doctor Powell's parsing of symptoms and determining an underlying diagnosis. From Eddie Mae I gained knowledge of how the gray handmaiden of loss may affect a person's health and how the doctor may provide comfort, not just with medicines or surgery, but also by the use of his or her personality. And from Nannette, I gaped red faced at a truly impressive set of boobs and gained an understanding of how physical appearance undergirds self-confidence.

Moreover, I experienced the excitement and affirmation that goes with practicing medicine. Wendell, Eddie Mae, and Nannette each provided Doctor Powell with intellectual challenges, testing both his experience and his knowledge. It dawned on me that medicine could provide these same benefits for me along with a similar stream of mostly appreciative patients. From August of 1962 onward, I never seriously considered any alternative to the field of medicine. Sorry, Mom and Dad.

So perhaps the time is long overdue to say thanks. Thank you, Doctor Bill Powell, for being my very first medical mentor. You were great. Thank you, too, hulking middle linebacker, for the opportune injury, even though my thumb hurt like hell. I also thank all the patients who tolerated my presence, and by so doing allowed me to gain life-changing insights that otherwise would have been missed.

And yes, thank you, too, Nannette, for providing an unforgettable, eye-popping experience. And allow me to share a final lesson learned from Nannette—size really does matter, and in women no less.

*Chapter 2*

# THE MIDNIGHT MEAL

*History doesn't repeat itself, but it sure does rhyme.*

—Mark Twain

The clock read five minutes till midnight—my favorite time of an intern's on-call day. All consults and admissions had been completed, the emergency room cleared, and the hospital tempo reduced from a flat-out gallop to a more leisurely trot. A comforting stillness settled over the "Old General."

The midnight meal was never sumptuous or fancy. It might consist of sandwiches, soup, and French fries from lunch; macaroni and cheese, green beans, and pork chops from dinner; and the ubiquitous lime Jell-O from who knows when. Still, twenty or so interns and residents along with a few medical students would converge each midnight on the hospital's cafeteria. Our jobs required a great expenditure of energy, hustling about in search of X-rays and lab reports, making rounds on patients, and working long hours in surgery and providing consultations—all of which created the need for middle-of-the-night nourishment. Camaraderie and emotional release also were on the menu. Perhaps more sustaining than the food, these informal gatherings maintained the high spirits of the house staff.

I entered the cafeteria at the magic hour on my first night on call, served myself a heaping plate of food, and took a seat. I felt mildly apprehensive, not knowing what to expect from the gathering of tired and rumpled house officers. I did not sit alone for long.

"Hello. Don Blossom, pedes resident." A lanky, casually dressed doctor stood before me, extending his hand. He folded himself into a seat next to me.

"Well, hi, I'm Tom Hutton, rotating intern."

"What service you on?" asked Don, as he began to devour a plate of meatballs, mixed salad, and fried potatoes.

"Newborn ICU with Strickland," I said while pounding out small crimson jets of ketchup onto my meatloaf.

"You'll love her, a fine teacher, knows her stuff." Don's blue eyes sparkled with mirth.

"Amazed how efficient her unit is, runs like an assembly line. Great nurses too, but nerve-wracking beginning on the NICU; little tykes get sick fast."

Don Blossom smiled, no doubt sensing my anxiety with the NICU, and finished chewing a large bite of Swedish meatball. He steepled his fingers and developed a thoughtful expression on his clean-shaven face. "Have spent two rotations in NICU; nurses are the greatest. I'd advise you to listen closely to what they say."

I nodded my head. "They're great," I said. Across the way I observed two intent interns with large spoons gouging into a large container of ice cream, looking like hungry bears pawing salmon from a stream.

"Doctor Strickland runs an informal but disciplined unit," Don said, looking at me intently. "Just don't piss her off."

Don described how Martha Strickland's personality changed when she became angry, and while rare, it was not a pretty sight. After first determining if I would be interested, he addressed a few practicalities about working within our out-of-date hospital.

"Avoid the elevators, antiquated and too slow. Got stuck for an hour once," said Don. "The whole time the hospital operator was paging me, her voice getting more and more shrill. Couldn't get out of the elevator to phone her for what she wanted."

"Guess this year I'll get my exercise on the stairs."

"Biggest hassle is lab work; lab is understaffed. Have to draw your own blood samples. Techs are overtaxed and get downright cranky," Don said with a shrug.

"Any shortcuts?" I asked.

"You might consider bribes. I've tried desserts from the cafeteria; works for some. Have resorted to chocolate for a couple of the more intransigent ones. I call it expanding their service mind-set by enlarging their waistlines." Don smiled broadly.

"Well, now, that's a thought." I was feeling pleased that Don Blossom had chosen to offer me his advice.

"One resident took to laying the wood to one of the techs, the one they call Vampire. Worked great for him while he was here but after he left, Vampire felt used and still tends to hold it against all white-coated men. I'm not sure what she was expecting, with him having a wife, three kids, a dog, and a mortgage."

"What about the old mustachioed fellow who runs the lab?" I asked.

"Peppermint schnapps, his weakness. Would give away his Polaris snowmobile for a regular supply of schnapps."

"I'll keep that in mind. Since I'm on a beer budget, don't know if I'll be buying any schnapps."

"One of the big problems around here is parking. House staff lot is three blocks down Chicago Avenue. Trust me, in January the trek is worthy of Ernest Shackelton. If no spot there, I've been known to walk over a mile to the hospital," Don said with a shudder. "Think Doctor Zhivago with icicles clinging to his mustache, not an enjoyable hike in the winter."

"Any suggestions for this warm weather intern?" I had been worried since my arrival in Minnesota after learning the winters not only were frigid but also had razor-sharp winds. Don might have noticed the concern on my face as he quickly responded.

"Well, just met you, but you seem a good sort." He looked around in a conspiratorial manner, leaned in, and said, "I put up a sign on the wall by the house staff parking lot. It read: reserved for medicine chief resident. It worked too. Few folks knew the chief resident never parked there—found an attending doctor who bused in and snatched his place in the nearby parking garage for staff physicians. I realized the chief resident's spot was not being used, but it needed to be, ahem, better identified. *Voil*à, the sign. Might want to check out the parking options for other chief residents from some of the other services."

The midnight meal also offered an informal way to obtain feedback from consulting doctors. Several months later and by fortunate circumstance working with Don Blossom on the pediatric service, I recall obtaining helpful curbside consults from the pulmonary and renal fellows.

"Looks like you guys got your hands full with the Sophie Mortensen case," said Clark Bennett, a burly, sandy-haired pulmonary fellow. I noticed his large Littmann stethoscope draped from his coat pocket looking like a tangled garden hose.

"Thanks for coming in the other night. Sophie was going down faster than the *Edmund Fitzgerald*." I had been impressed by how skillfully Clark Bennett had slipped the small airway through her voice box into Sophie's trachea. Under much pressure, successfully performing the feat, I thought, was akin to hitting a nail head with a .22 at one hundred yards.

Harvey Reasoner, a nephrology fellow, held court at an adjacent metal, white-topped rectangular table. He too had consulted on Sophie, whom he knew was monopolizing our time with her exchange transfusions.

"How're her kidneys doing?" asked Harvey, a burly ex-football player from the University of Michigan.

"Kidneys still holding up," I replied. I went on to provide him with the latest measures of kidney function. This led to a discussion of what degree of abnormality would prompt us to begin dialysis. Harvey identified several additional potential concerns, as if I needed more to worry about. Nevertheless, these informal exchanges at the midnight meal were always easier to understand than the turgid, handwritten, and nearly illegible consultations filed in the patients' charts.

Not just business was discussed at the midnight meal. Funny anecdotes were often shared. Stories that involved drunken faculty physicians doing things like polkaing with napkins draped over their heads at hospital parties were particularly well received.

Even though the house staff and attending physicians worked well together, the house staff envied the better-paid attending physicians. Given that dynamic, stories of the attending physicians' periodic abject business failures were always welcome as well. We house staff, on the other hand, assumed when we reached that stage in our careers we would magically gain shrewd business acumen and enhanced financial prudence.

A favorite topic at each midnight meal was the latest and most inconvenient structural or machine failure at the Old General. To no one's surprise, the hospital, while passing the white-glove test for cleanliness, was becoming ever creakier in its operations. The Old General and the neighboring private Metropolitan Medical Center were slated to merge into a spanking-new facility. Because of this planned consolidation, little money was being expended for upkeep on the soon-to-be-destroyed old hospital.

A popular discussion among the male house officers surrounded our female comrades. Good leads were traded like prized fishing spots as to which nurses would most easily shed their white frocks.

"Did you hear about the cardiology fellow and OR nurse buffing the operating table?" asked radiology resident Todd Lewis one evening. "Yup, right there on the stainless steel. Brandy must have a thing for masks, because both were as naked as the day they were born except for surgical masks. Humping away like crazed weasels they were. What they overlooked in their passion was the surveillance camera. Filmed what must have been their very cold act of copulation. Yep, caught the whole episode, *en flagrante*. I've seen it, too. Folks in radiology refer to the video as 'Hank the Hammer Meets Brandy-fucking Nightingale.' Jack from hospital security gave me a private showing—swapped it for his barium GI series. His little ulcer really paid off."

All the guffawing provided emotional release at the end of many a tense day. The joking, the mutual support, and the affirmation of medical judgments, not yet cemented by lengthy experience, made the challenges somehow more tolerable.

Practical help for my personal monetary shortage also came my way at the midnight meal. I had heard that Pat Olsen, the chief resident in the emergency room, was quite the entrepreneur. Olsen usually had a number of interns surrounding him, as he represented the gateway to profitable moonlighting. My opportunity to approach him finally arose at a late meal in the form of an empty chair next to him.

"Pat, what's it take to ride the ambulance?" I asked.

"Not a problem. Let me know when you're available, and I'll assign you a night or two a month," he replied casually. He said this while referring to a small scheduling booklet he always kept in his rear pocket.

"Great and thanks," I said.

"Say, Hutton, you know anything about hockey?" he asked. I had learned from other interns that Olsen regularly scheduled doctors to work the high school hockey games and that the pay was good.

"Sure, I know hockey," I lied. With a pregnant wife and a light paycheck, I felt situational ethics were called for in that particular exchange.

"Can let you work hockey games, if you want. Good money, not much to it."

For reasons I never understood, the ever-cautious Minnesota Legislature had passed a law requiring a doctor's presence at every high school hockey game. What actual benefit I provided that year, shuffling across the ice with my black medical bag to check the status of a downed player, was questionable. Nevertheless the one hundred dollars per match came in handy. Thank you, Minnesota Legislature, for this act of welfare for financially struggling interns.

I later lost track of Pat. Given his excellent business sense, I suspect by now he is running a chain of hospitals, or a large group practice, or at the very least an extensive chain of highly profitable imaging centers.

When reminiscing about the early 1970s, I am amazed how the technology and practice of medicine have evolved from those days. Some of today's modern imaging techniques and therapeutic achievements were unimaginable at the time of my internship. Now smartphones, Google and Medline searches, and electronic medical records make important information readily available.

The practice of medicine has become more sophisticated and data driven. These wonderful technological devices have as an unfortunate byproduct, reduced human-to-human transfer of information. This makes it possible for physicians to spend less time with colleagues and more time with their devices. I fear what may occur if this impersonalization is taken to its logical end.

This is not to imply the newer advances are unimportant or fail to elevate the quality of medicine; they certainly do. It is only that the midnight meal and other physician-to-physician interactions provided crucial social lubrication, important for providing good health care and for smoothing physician relations. Such interactions gave us an opportunity for physician mutual support, an encouragement never offered by even the most "user-friendly" machines.

Some would claim the midnight meal has become an anachronism of an earlier medical age, much like the black bag I carried to the last day of my medical practice. I respectfully disagree with this opinion. In addition to providing a human interface among physicians, the quaint custom of the midnight meal also erected a bulwark against veering too far afield into a numbers-crunching, overly compartmentalized, and hyperspecialized medicine.

Absent this ritual, some means will be needed in the future to maintain doctor networking and to foster collegiality. The practice of medicine is, in the final analysis, a human-to-human transfer and rendering of care. The art of medicine with its need for good listening and speaking is as important as the increasingly technological aspects of the profession.

Good communication among physicians will, to a substantial degree, determine future efficiencies and promote the rendering of excellent health care. It will also govern the all-important improvement in safety and quality—the holy grail of our evolving American health-care system.

## Chapter 3

# TRANSFUSIONS

*Faith is daring the soul to go beyond what the eyes can see.*

—William Newton Clark

*Hope sees the invisible, feels the unimaginable*
*And achieves the impossible.*

—Anonymous

**Day 1: 8:57 a.m.**

While I sat in the emergency room, puzzling over lab values from an earlier patient, I heard squeaking sounds from a tatty metal gurney. This interrupted my thoughts as it raced by me toward the ambulance bay. This all-too-frequent event inevitably prompted tightness in the pits of stomachs of the emergency room personnel, especially wet-behind-the-ears interns like me. The place was the ER of the Hennepin County General Hospital in early winter, 1972, and it was a beehive of activity. Strobe lights from the ambulance flashed eerily down the hallway. On making my way down the corridor, I saw a burly, white-clad man lower the side rail of the gurney and from the ambulance scoop up in his arms a tiny form and gently lay her on the wheeled stretcher.

A week earlier young Sophie Mortensen had made her Christmas list. She had twice listed a specific doll along with a paint set, a dollhouse, and a new pink dress. While Sophie sat at her small child's desk double-checking her list, Sophie's mother noticed her flushed cheeks and wondered if Sophie might be falling ill—suspicions later borne out when the girl developed fever, generalized droopiness, and the telltale spots of chicken-pox.

Sophie had been recovering from chickenpox until a day before her arrival in the ER. Overnight she had suffered nausea and repeated vomiting. To her parents' dismay, the following morning Sophie was difficult to arouse and babbling nonsensically. Her frantic parents summoned an ambulance and directed the driver to race to the General Hospital in Minneapolis, a teaching hospital for the University of Minnesota.

**Day 1: 9:03 a.m.**

As the intern rotating on pediatrics, I received the call from the emergency room to admit this incoming patient. The blue-eyed, six-year-old Sophie Mortensen, as if in a fitful sleep, soon arrived in a curtained room in the ER. The staff carefully transferred her from the gurney to a more comfortable adjacent bed.

The saucy laboratory technician nicknamed Vampire by the interns swooped in and drew several tubes of blood. Simultaneously, a nurse inserted a second intravenous line and connected it to an overhead bottle of fluid. An EKG (electrocardiogram) technician placed leads for a heart tracing. A radiology technician slid a film under the child for a chest X-ray. I positioned myself within this beehive of workers to examine this very sick little girl.

"Sophie, open your eyes!" I pleaded, gaining no response.

"Squeeze my fingers!" Again, nothing.

Sophie thrashed at her sheet, as if mindlessly shooing away flies. Moving aside golden curls from her forehead revealed several partially healed pox marks. These small imperfections marred what otherwise was a creamy, soft complexion. Her breathing, at thirty breaths per minute, was far too rapid and sounded like a miniature steam engine. When I struck the tendons just below Sophie's knees to check her reflexes, her lower legs jumped too briskly. I gently probed beneath the right side of her rib cage and felt an unmistakably enlarged liver, extending a good two fingerbreadths below her delicate rib cage.

Within fifteen minutes the laboratory called with her stat lab test results. These values revealed a low blood sugar, prolonged blood clotting studies, and abnormal liver tests. I contacted Don Blossom, my pediatric resident, to discuss this constellation of unusual lab findings.

While only three years older than I, Don struck me as a grizzled, battle-scarred veteran. In my brief time on pediatrics, he had proven remarkably knowledgeable but also affable, approachable, and a good teacher. He was lanky and moved with the fluidity of a basketball player. At times suffused by a veritable storm of problems, Don always could be counted on to remain unflappable. I found his attitude calming for my own surging emotions.

I headed for the nearest telephone and asked the operator to page Doctor Blossom.

"Don, I'm in the ER and am baffled."

"What's up, Tom?"

I provided the physical findings and laboratory results. Don absorbed the information without comment and asked a few questions before responding.

"Sounds like she may have Reye's syndrome," Don said.

"Reye's syndrome?" I knew Reye's to be a serious childhood illness but was otherwise largely unfamiliar with the diagnosis. "I know we discussed that in med school, but I don't remember the details. Can you fill me in?"

"It's fairly unusual—typically follows mild infections and causes liver failure, clotting abnormalities, and brain swelling."

"How bad is it?" I asked.

"Very serious with substantial mortality. Order a blood ammonia value. It's a measure for how well the liver is working.

Also obtain spinal fluid for routine analysis to rule out encephalitis. May take several hours but these should pin down the diagnosis."

Over the prolonged hospital stay that would later unfold, I learned much about the Mortensen family. James and Francine Mortensen, Sophie's parents, lived in a tidy, buttoned-down suburb southwest of Minneapolis. They were a handsome couple, smartly dressed, nicely groomed, and well educated. They did not represent the typical clientele for the inner-city Hennepin County General Hospital.

James owned a successful, medium-size construction business. While his workload took him away from home ten to twelve hours a day, and often days at a time, he always carved out time for outings with their children and for school activities.

Francine, or Franny as her husband and friends called her, stayed busy as a homemaker and the principal parent for Sophie and Bobby, the latter a twelve-year-old athletically minded boy. She volunteered as a tutor at the children's school and also with a mission group at her church. I often observed a modest silver cross hanging from Franny's neck.

James and Franny struck me, even from our earliest conversations, as nurturing parents.

Their daughter's strange illness naturally terrified them. James tried to remain stoic, yet an occasionally tremulous voice gave evidence of his anxiety. Franny often searched beseechingly the faces of the doctors and nurses with penetrating brown eyes. She pled, "Please do all you can for our little Sophie."

**Day 1: 11:10 a.m.**
Sophie lay dwarfed by the large bed. Intravenous tubing and monitoring wires extended from her small body like tentacles of an octopus. Connie Baker, the charge nurse on pediatrics, hurried toward me with a piece of paper fluttering in her outstretched hand. Connie impressed me as having the mental toughness to endure the hectic routine and the overwhelming compassion necessary for a pediatric nurse. I admired her greatly.

"Call from the lab on Sophie Mortensen."

I scanned the results. The spinal fluid tests were negative for encephalitis with no white blood cells found in the sample. The blood ammonia level was elevated, showing her liver's inability to metabolize that bodily toxin. These findings provided still stronger evidence for acute liver failure and confirmed Don's diagnosis of Reye's syndrome.

"Thanks, Connie, I'll let Doctor Blossom know." As usual, Don had been spot on.

**Day 1: Afternoon**
Sophie worsened. She briefly became agitated and then stopped moving altogether. Reflexes that measure brain-stem functions became sluggish and her body's functions were winding down like a failing battery-operated clock. Her pupils dilated and became poorly reactive to a bright light. When I stimulated Sophie by lightly strumming on her breastbone, she demonstrated a disturbing neurological posturing of her arms and legs. Her slender arms flexed with bulging biceps, as if trying to intimidate the disease that stalked her young life. Sophie was desperately ill and inexorably worsening with every passing hour. Her deterioration proved momentarily too agonizing to watch.

I averted my eyes, peering out the window to the traffic moving below on Chicago Avenue. The corridor along which traffic crawled had been narrowed by snow that was now piled high along both sides of the road. The movement and occasional jockeying for position among the cars reassured me of robust life forces. The very normality of the scene and lack of awareness of Sophie's crisis reminded me that for most, everyday life went on unchanged.

**Day 1: 7:00 p.m.**
Although required to leave her bedside to care for other patients, I returned frequently to check on Sophie. On each visit, I found James and Franny helicoptering near the bed.

"How's she doing?" I asked.

"Well, not restless but still not saying anything," Franny whispered, as if wishing not to wake a sleeping Sophie. Although she looked as if she were asleep, I knew Sophie balanced precariously on the thin knife's edge between life and death.

I reexamined the young patient. Again she had worsened. No doubt, a strained look appeared on my face.

"Now, Doctor Hutton, we know you're doing everything you can. We've been praying for you and Doctor Blossom," James said.

Her parents just then bowed their heads and silently began to pray. Despite their worry and grief, both maintained upbeat attitudes. I was struck by how their faith sustained them during this ordeal.

Within ten hours of the onset of Sophie's delirium, all treatments had been brought to bear on her liver failure, clotting abnormalities, electrolyte imbalance, and brain swelling. Little was left to do except reexamine, wait, hope, and along with James and Franny—pray.

**Day 1: Midnight**
That night Don and I pulled call. It was a long and difficult night. We stayed busy admitting sick children from the emergency room and attending children on the wards with spiking fevers, asthma attacks, and seizures. We also were called to see two "squirters," neonates with explosive diarrhea. Although these cases warranted hospitalization in order to maintain adequate hydration, they were in no way as serious as the illness from Sophie suffered.

Periodically throughout the long night one of us would return to check on Sophie. Her findings remained discouraging, as she continued her relentless downhill progression.

**Day 2: 3:00 a.m.**
Sophie's pupils had stopped reacting to light and her breathing had become uneven and irregular. The abnormal posturing of her extremities changed and acquired an even more dire neurological significance. With physical stimulation her arms now

straightened and stiffened and her tiny fists rotated repeatedly inward, as if digging a shallow grave.

"Time to tube her. Respirations need support," Don said.

A pulmonary doctor placed a small tube down her windpipe, inflated the cuff around the tracheal tube, and connected her to a ventilator.

"You think she'll survive, Don?" I asked out of earshot of her parents.

"Don't think so; doubt Sophie's going to make it." He said this with a grim look of resignation.

"Hell, just doesn't seem fair. She's so young—such a good family."

"Not much fair about dying, especially with children," Don said soberly.

### Day 2: 4:00 p.m.

I saw Don Blossom striding down the hallway, his white coat flapping and a medical journal tucked beneath his arm. I headed for the nurse's station to intercept him. Don's face radiated excitement.

"I've been in the library reading up on newer treatments for Reye's syndrome."

"Find something?"

"Well, I think so. In some cases exchange transfusions help."

This took several moments to register. "You mean we drain her blood?"

"Well, yes, but slowly, and in very small amounts at a time. Then we replace it with fresh blood," Don said patiently.

"You think it's our best chance, don't you."

"I do. It may be our only one. We need to talk to the parents and determine if they are willing to give it a try," Don replied. "The treatment will take hours, four or five at least. You up for it? Know we're pretty beat up after last night, but considering the alternative of doing nothing," and his voice trailed off.

"Let's go."

**Day 2: 4:10 p.m.**

Don Blossom swept toward Sophie's bed with me quick-stepping along beside. Her parents sat nearby. We approached and Don paused briefly at the bedside, gathering his thoughts.

"Mr. and Mrs. Mortensen, there's just no way to sugarcoat this. Sophie's worse despite everything we have tried," Don said earnestly.

"We feared that," said James. We trained our gazes on the motionless, beautiful little girl with the golden locks in the bed before us.

I added, "The results of Sophie's brain-wave test are back. Unfortunately, it's not good either." The test showed Sophie's brain waves were severely abnormal. The medical literature predicted Reye's patients with her abnormal EEG (electro-encephalogram) uniformly died. But Don and I had elected not to share this grim prognosis, believing it speculative and too dismal.

"I uncovered some recent medical literature that found exchange transfusions helpful," Don said. He went on to share more information about the improved outcome of Reye's patients who had undergone this procedure. He also gave other potential benefits as well as risks of the procedure. Don's presentation sounded hopeful, speculative, and at times fueled by desperation. Given the condition of Sophie, I feared the choice we gave the parents was really not an option at all—a real Hobson's choice.

I saw expectant looks exchanged between the parents and watched as their fear turned to hope. Almost in unison, they endorsed our plan with what I interpreted as more hope than expectation. Within minutes blood was sent to the laboratory for typing and cross matching.

Don and I then began to plan how to carry out the transfusions.

"Not enough room to work here," Don said.

"What about moving Sophie to the procedure room. It's not being used and the room is larger," I suggested.

Knowing the process would be slow and that Sophie would be temporarily unavailable to them, we convinced the parents to go home for some much-needed rest. We promised to contact them if problems arose during the night.

**Day 2: 10:00 p.m.**
Due to delays in matching the blood, the exchange transfusion did not begin until ten o'clock the second night. Don and I hung around the hospital catching up on charting, trying to hasten the blood-matching process, and keeping active in an attempt to stay awake.

At one point during the evening I overheard an irritated Don on the phone urging the lab technician, "Now come on, Vampire, surely you've matched the blood on Sophie Mortensen by now." I then saw a startled look on Don's face as he removed the phone from his ear and stared quizzically at the dead phone line.

"One call too many?" I asked.

**Day 2: 11:10 p.m.**
The exchange transfusion, once started, proved laborious. We would remove a measure of Sophie's blood from a large catheter and through another replace it with an equal portion of fresh blood. The idea was to remove the ammonia and other toxins from Sophie's bloodstream. The in and out of the procedure grew monotonous. *Pull, push, pull, push, pull, push. . . .* Both of us were intermittently nodding off even as we stood, leaning against her bed. We finished the procedure around 4:30 a.m. Exhausted, Don and I swapped uncertain smiles and headed home for brief, long-overdue rest.

**Day 3: 8:15 a.m.**
Reexamination of Sophie found her liver more enlarged. I felt it extending five fingerbreadths below her lower rib with a distinct firmness like shoe leather. Except for her metabolic condition, she remained at a neurological level that would meet the

definition of brain death. Her muscles were flaccid. Her pupils remained nonreactive when a bright light was directed at them, and she demonstrated no spontaneous breathing.

Her tenuous existence depended on her brain stem, and it was slowly dying. Within this most primitive portion of her brain resided the most basic life forces of breathing and regulation of heart rate.

At the top of the brain stem sat the thalamus, the part of the brain that includes a tiny gland called the pineal. Descartes, centuries before, had described the pineal gland as the site of the soul. This tiny gland and the remainder of Sophie's brain stem were being suffocated by this soul-choking, lethal illness.

"At least her ammonia is down. It's hopeful," Don said. His body language belied his more positive statement.

"Guess we better update the parents," I suggested.

We visited Sophie's parents, who had changed their clothes and appeared somewhat refreshed after their brief time at home. Don began the update, and I stood silently by his side, feeling like Sancho Panza to his Don Quixote.

"Everything went fine last night with the exchange transfusion. Sophie's ammonia level is lower this morning. Otherwise, she is about the same."

As ever the parents remained supportive and appreciative of our efforts despite Sophie's poor condition.

"Our whole church is praying," Franny said. James and Franny went on to tell us that prayer chains had been formed, not only throughout their own congregation, but also throughout the greater church membership. Sophie was receiving countless prayers from prayer warriors across the nation.

I perceived these collective spiritual acts provided Franny and James a renewed sense of confidence and hope. In a strange way, I felt my own resolve strengthening with a growing aspiration that Sophie somehow must not be allowed to die.

**Day 3: 11:15 a.m.**
By late morning the ammonia level again had crept upward to scary heights. Don's medical literature urged repeated exchange

transfusions to maintain the ammonia levels within a certain range, so that by midday we had begun another blood exchange. All went smoothly with Don and me working silently and efficiently. *Pull, push, pull, push, pull, push.* . . .

**Day 3: 8:00 p.m.**
Late admissions to our pediatrics service kept us busy late into the day, admitting sick children and writing orders. Around 8:00 p.m., I received an overhead page from Don. Sophie's recent ammonia level was again quite elevated. *This Reye's disease, like the hydra of Greek mythology, presents one attack after another.* Don told me his most recent examination found Sophie moribund.

**Day 3: 8:10 p.m.**
Don and I arrived at the bedside at the same time. James and Franny sat prayerfully alongside the bed.

"I don't know what else we can offer," Don said. "Her condition just isn't responding. We've done everything we know to do."

Results from the second EEG had returned with the same grim prediction, namely that she would not recover. On this occasion, we shared the bad prognosis with the parents.

"Things just continue to get worse and worse," Don said.

The dejected silence that followed was punctuated by the continuous mechanical wheezing of the ventilator. After an extended pause, their gazes moved from searching each other's face to studying the faces of Don and me.

Franny began speaking in a tentative way. "We understand you've done everything you know to do. And we appreciate how hard you've worked." Her voice was plaintive and sorrowful.

"Are there any questions we can try to answer?" I asked, trying to momentarily break the sadness.

"Please, just don't give up," said James. He emitted a muffled sob with his words. "We know the power of prayer. We're sure, as convinced as we can be, that Sophie will get well. We feel God's healing spirit in our hearts."

**Day 3: 8:30 p.m.**

As Don and I left the ward, he asked me to join him in the cafeteria. The cafeteria was empty, as our arrival was midway between dinnertime and the house officers' midnight meal. We pulled out two chairs across the table from each other, slumped down, and leaned dejectedly forward with heads almost touching.

"I wish I had the Mortensens' faith that Sophie's going to improve," Don said.

"Me too. Incredible how earnest they are and how their faith maintains their hope. You think she has any chance?"

"Slim and none. It's looking really grim."

At this juncture both of us must have appeared and certainly felt exhausted. Our spirits sagged. To try so hard, yet have the beautiful little Sophie inescapably worsen before our eyes—it was difficult to bear. Notes of discouragement riddled our conversation. Finally, Don lifted his eyes from the table and began to speak softly and tentatively.

"Tom, I know it's a lot to ask, but are you willing to give it one more shot? Probably means us pulling another all-nighter. Can't pass this train wreck onto the on-call team. They're just too busy to take this one on."

"Don't even need to ask. I'll do whatever it takes to help that little girl." I knew Don had a little girl of his own, just a few years younger than Sophie. My determination was fortified knowing my own child grew within Trudy's womb. He too could face such a horrible event, and I knew how desperately I would want everything possible done.

**Day 3: 9:00 p.m.**

We walked back to Sophie's bedside. We shared with the parents our thoughts about one final exchange transfusion. Slight smiles spread across their faces.

"We felt confident you'd come up with something. James and I prayed about it and know the good Lord heard us. Bless you both, we know you're so tired," said Franny.

**Day 3: 11:45 p.m.**

That night Don and I performed another exchange transfusion. Again out came blood with its impurities and in went the fresh blood. In and out, in and out, throughout the long night we pulled and pushed our large syringes like slow-moving pistons, all the time hoping to expunge the foul elements that made Sophie so ill. Around 4:00 a.m. we finished. We nodded at each other, too tired to even speak. After asking the nurses to call us at 7:00 for morning rounds, Don and I stumbled off to our on-call rooms.

**Day 4**

Something miraculous occurred the following day and continued on gradually over the next days and weeks. I am still at a loss to explain it. To a nonscientist it would be called a miracle. To a medical scientist, the treatments must have finally worked and the body, given a respite from the toxins, managed to heal.

Over the next day Sophie's coma became lighter. Not long afterward, her pupils began to react to light, as if her eyes had again adjusted to perceiving the beauty of the world. Her ability to sit improved, along with her ability to swallow, smell, hear, and visually track. When I checked her lab report, I found her ammonia values to have fallen to normal. *Normal!* I felt beyond incredulous. I could not restrain myself and, while reviewing the lab work, jumped up from my chair and yelled, "Wahoo," prompting disapproving but tolerant smiles from a group of nearby nurses.

Within days we removed Sophie from the ventilator. Her breathing became deep and even like a metronome. She began to move her arms and legs, at first without purpose, then with clearer intent. Eventually she awakened and began to speak.

She opened her azure eyes, fixed on her parents, and said, "Hi, Mommy. Hi, Daddy." As I viewed this scene, I was greatly affected and felt tears escape my eyes. I rapidly turned away.

**Day 31**

One month after coming into the hospital, Sophie extended her arms upward to hug the necks of her doctors and nurses. Many wet eyes watched as Sophie walked hand-in-hand with her smiling parents out of the pediatrics ward. Her memory and coordination were destined slowly to improve.

Before departing, Franny turned, cleared her throat, and spoke: "God bless you all." Her warm eyes and smile overflowed with grateful emotion. She blew a kiss to all those assembled. When Franny attempted further words, they failed her. Yet we all knew she needed to say nothing else. We all knew the remarkable event that we had witnessed and felt overwhelmingly grateful for the successful outcome.

James stepped forward and said, "We'll never forget what you did for our Sophie." I noticed his ruddy cheeks glistened.

The doctors and nurses waved stoically, sniffing back their tears. Not a head turned away as the family walked out of the pediatrics ward. After losing sight of them, each doctor and nurse reluctantly did the required mental pivot toward other waiting tasks.

**Nine Months Later**

At Sophie's appointment nine months later, she was dressed in a checked jumper and white blouse, with red ribbons in her shoulder-length golden blond hair. Sophie had grown one and a half inches and had gained ten pounds. Of greater importance, Sophie's speech and thinking appeared wonderfully normal. According to her proud parents, she was performing at the top of her class. This incredible outcome exceeded my wildest expectations.

For years even after moving away from Minneapolis, I received short notes from Franny, usually around Christmastime. Often she would enclose pictures of Sophie. I learned Sophie continued to perform successfully in school and placed at the top of her class. I learned her favorite subjects, her enjoyment of Brownies and then Girl Scouts, and her enjoyment of dancing. Years later I learned of Sophie having developed an interest in music, and her hope one day to study music at the University of Minnesota.

Once with mock consternation, one of Franny's letters reported that Sophie, by then in early adolescence and with hormones flooding her system, had discovered boys. An accompanying photo showed that the little girl I had known years before had grown into a lovely young woman. The picture showed not only a lovely Sophie, but also a face bearing an inquisitive, lively, and playful expression.

I did not know then, nor was I ever to know, to what extent Don's and my efforts had contributed to Sophie's survival. But Franny's convictions over the years never flagged. At the end of each note, Franny always gave thanks to Doctor Blossom and me, crediting us with saving young Sophie's life. Franny wrote she knew the Lord placed us at the General Hospital to assist in healing Sophie. Our presence, she said, was no mere accident.

Sometime after my family and I moved to Texas in 1981, I lost track of Sophie and her parents. But I shall, for the rest of my life, never lose them from my memory. The Mortensen family will occupy a special chamber tucked deep within my heart.

To this day, I do not fully understand what pulled Sophie through those desperate hours and drama-filled days. While a believer, I have always assumed that once God established order, he pretty much backed off, leaving mankind to operate with free will.

Given Sophie's extraordinary outcome, I would never discount James and Franny's view of a more direct and personal involvement from on high. I am tempted to speculate that the exchange transfusions addressed more than just toxins. It is as if Sophie received infusions of hope and prayer from countless, anonymous supporters and possibly, just possibly, infusions of inspired and divine intervention.

*Chapter 4*

# LEARNING CURVE

*"You can't smooth out the surf but you can learn to ride the waves."*

—Author unknown

Like an aging queen with her bulging midriff and fleshy arms spread in welcoming gesture, the Hennepin County General Hospital squatted in downtown Minneapolis on the corner of Fifth Street and Portland Avenue. The skyline had over the years extended upward, dwarfing the old hospital. With its crumbling building, the Old General was living medicine in a dying facility. A thing of architectural beauty, she was not. In 1972 few would recognize the old brick building with its sooty gray exterior for what it was: a magnificent incubator for young doctors and an excellent provider of high-quality health care.

The hospital began in 1887 as the Minneapolis City Hospital. The initial two-hundred-bed East Wing was built in 1901. When I arrived, it housed numerous patient wards as well as the interns' sleeping quarters. The original building had actually been pleasing to the eye, with tall Greek columns gracing its main entrance. But by the time I arrived, its pillars and gargoyles had required patching and plastering and the façade appeared ready to fall down.

With the Great Depression had come diminished public

funding. Necessity over the years drove development of eight additional boxlike buildings, and by the 1970s all of the additions were in an advanced state of decay. About these add-ons it can only be said they were functional and had briefly relieved the hospital's overcrowded conditions.

When I began my internship July 1, 1972, I learned what the hospital lacked in physical presence, it more than made up for in *esprit de corps*, efficient management, and excellent health care. I felt fortunate to have successfully competed for an intern position at the Old General and was eager to get the year under way.

Physicians have often described their internships as the best

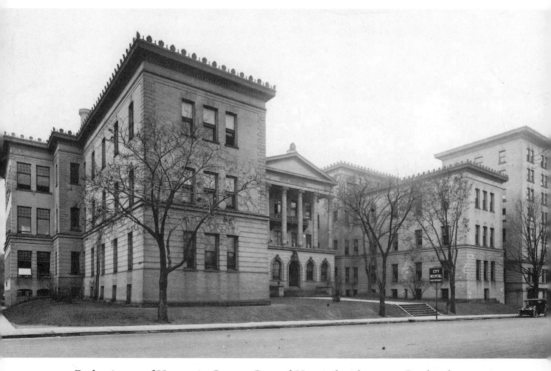

Early picture of Hennepin County General Hospital with ornate Greek columns at main entrance of hospital. By the time I arrived in 1972, the building had become thoroughly decrepit, but the hospital provided excellent health care and served as an incubator for many "baby docs." (Used by permission of Hennepin County Medical Center Museum)

year in their careers. I agree, although I constantly verged on complete physiological exhaustion.

In addition to the remarkable Sophie Mortensen, three clinical vignettes from the year stand out in my memory. I share them here.

**July 1, 8:05 a.m.**
Before me, looking like a diapered gnome, lay the tiniest baby I had ever seen. At just two pounds and one ounce, Baby Boy Pederson's pale, translucent skin had the appearance of a china doll. I was expected to provide this smidgen of protoplasm with nutrition, ventilator management, and ongoing treatment. At first I worried about even lifting or turning the baby from side to side for fear of breaking him.

Day one of my internship and there I stood, staring blankly into the incubator. My initial reaction was numbness. Several long moments passed before I fully understood that this tyke depended on me as much as he had earlier depended on his placenta. Dry-mouthed anxiety engulfed me like a hot desert wind.

My thoughts returned to the prior week, when ironically I had confided in Trudy, my homesick-for-Texas wife, that I felt prepared for my internship, so long as I started on an adult service, preferably with chronic patients.

"Adults don't go sour as quickly as kids, and they can tell you where it hurts," I had said. I would have been satisfied with *any* service so long as it was not pediatrics.

Yet, on my very first day of internship, not only did I find myself ensconced in the pediatrics service but also assigned, as if by some sadist, to the neonatal intensive care unit (NICU). My earlier confidence had dissipated like smoke before a fan. I had little practical experience with children of any age, much less these fragile babies. I felt ill prepared and frightened.

The NICU was built in sections starting in 1914 and looked every minute of its age. Its flat roof of asphalt and gravel sagged and leaked. The annex had connecting tunnels and corridors that proved tricky to travel because of stored beds jammed together up against the walls, leaving only a narrow center passageway. A large hole in the wall of the NICU exposed what had once been a leaking pipe. Like much of the old hospital, undone repairs pleaded for unavailable resources.

Across the NICU I spotted my newest mentor, Doctor Martha Strickland, director of the NICU. This diminutive woman surveyed her unit like a mother hen watching over her chicks. Her experienced gaze never missed a thing. She would prove to be a superb teacher and role model.

Scurrying among the incubators were four efficient ladies in white. I watched them begin intravenous lines, feed babies, hang tiny infusions of medicine, and change diapers. To this inexperienced rookie, they appeared as white-smocked wizards. I determined to ingratiate myself to them by whatever means possible, knowing that without their help I was in big, big trouble.

On that first day, Doctor Strickland gathered her three new and fidgety interns and explained to us our duties. She introduced us to the nurses and assigned our babies. Doctor Strickland demonstrated how to examine such tiny infants and how to perform certain minor procedures. The activity and mental focus helped to tamp down my simmering anxiety.

Mercifully, the first few days passed without incident. I scrutinized the actions of the nurses for their techniques and asked many questions of Doctor Strickland. The nurses answered my queries and helped me whenever needed. At times they would approach we new interns for medical orders. If in response to their questions they encountered a dull stare like that of a cow chewing her cud, they tactfully would whisper what we should write. I knew this was the nurses' unit and that I was a mere transient within it. MD degree or not, their experience trumped my recently awarded status of physician.

**July 8, 9:00 a.m.**
One morning a nurse approached me. "Doctor Strickland wants you to do the new-baby examinations on the three newbies," said

Gretchen, a green-eyed, mid-twenty-year-old, scarlet-haired nurse. "Said she'd be back in a couple of hours, some important meeting in the pedes department at the U."

"I'm on it—well, as soon as I get this danged IV started. Need a magnifying glass to even find these minuscule veins," I complained. I noticed my thumb was equal in size to the preemie's entire hand.

In a few minutes, Gretchen slipped the teensy IV needle into the baby's vein, taped it in place, and started the infusion. I then moved on to the new-baby exams. I removed the first baby from his incubator and placed him under the heat lamps.

The first two exams went without incident and I felt myself becoming more efficient in my task. Only a fraction of the time was needed to examine an infant as compared to an adult, simply because there was not much to auscultate, palpate, and inspect. I jotted down my chart notes and moved on to baby number three.

Baby Boy Selness was batting third in the lineup that morning. He weighed in at a whopping four pounds, nine ounces, a virtual giant for the NICU, the land of preemies. Despite being premature, his lungs had functioned well, avoiding the necessity for a ventilator. While smaller than the average newborn, he appeared robust, well formed, and as if he simply needed time to grow.

I began my exam by peering into his ears with a miniature ear speculum attached to my otoscope. I palpated his little belly and listened with my stethoscope to his heart and lungs. As I removed his diaper and turned to lay it on a nearby shelf, an entirely unexpected event occurred. A loud popping noise startled me, causing me to spin my head back forcefully. An explosion had scattered bits of lightbulb glass. Instantaneously, the luminance had diminished. I attempted to blink away the objectionable scene, but my blinking was to no avail, and I was forced to recognize that hot shards of glass had sprayed over the counter and, most critically, the baby. The child immediately began to wail.

My world compressed. I began frantically to pick off hot

glass from the baby's delicate skin. Beneath the glass, I observed small red blemishes—first-degree burns. My heart pounded. I felt my face flush. The baby by this time was bawling louder still.

I had the presence of mind to search the baby's mouth for stray bits of glass. I found none. Soon I sensed Gretchen at my side. She captured the significance of the situation almost immediately. Using a paper towel, Gretchen began calmly sweeping pieces of glass from the exam area into a wastebasket that she held to the side of the counter.

*This woman must have ice water in her veins.*

"What a trick shot," Gretchen said in a calm and measured voice.

"What do you mean?" I said.

"Well, little Wild Bill Hickok here hit that bulb from a distance of over three feet," Gretchen said in her matter-of-fact voice. "That's quite an aim for the tyke, and apparently hit it with the force of a fire hose."

I had been distracted placing the diaper and had not observed the little fellow's prodigious urinary feat.

*So that's why the heat lamp exploded.*

"Can't trust these little guys; girls are easier. Soon as the guys slip their diapers, they let it fly. Trust me, learned the hard way," she said, giving her face a mock wipe with the back of her hand and flicking her scarlet hair.

Gretchen and I finished searching for additional burns to which we applied ointment. None appeared severe enough to require bandaging. I worried whether the baby might have more serious, unobserved injuries. I barely noticed my own burned fingers, acquired by removing hot glass from the baby, or the burns on my forearms, so keenly focused was I on my task.

*On the job a week and already a burned baby. What's Doctor Strickland going to think? How will the mother react?*

Gretchen's positive attitude and ongoing light banter kept my spirits from sinking too far into despair.

*Might she know something else I don't?*

When Doctor Strickland returned to the NICU later that morning, I took a deep, calming breath and resolutely approached her. I believed it best to immediately share the bad news.

I had learned useful information about Doctor Strickland from Don Blossom, the friendly pediatric resident who sat with me at an earlier midnight meal. He said that while she was far from physically intimidating, when angered, Doctor Strickland could develop the personality of a badger with a toothache. At that moment I was feeling heartsick over Baby Boy Selness. My sagging ego would have been easier to target than would an elephant trussed to a tree.

I explained what had happened and mentally cringed, fearing an incoming verbal fusillade. I felt my muscles tighten and my heart begin to pound. The outburst, mercifully, never came.

"Told them this would happen," Doctor Strickland said simply without even raising her voice. "Put in the work order three months ago, but Maintenance never found time to shield the babies from exploding heat lamps. Inevitable it was. Just a matter of time and male hydraulics."

I was relieved. It was clear I was not to be skewered and served up as a sacrificial lamb. But I still fretted over the baby's welfare. Doctor Strickland walked over to Baby Boy Selness's incubator and examined him. She assured me that the burns were minor and would heal without a trace. On hearing this, I exhaled a deep and pent-up sigh of relief.

Despite my absolution, I confess that Baby Boy Selness received close attention from me from then until the moment he transferred out of NICU to the newborn nursery. His gracious mother also accepted my explanation and heartfelt apology with surprising grace, leaving me to ponder how truly forgiving and wonderful people can be.

After a few weeks, the work in the NICU unbelievably began to feel routine. Nevertheless, I felt immense relief on finishing that first month's rotation. Dealing with ill preemies was like a circus act of keeping ever-increasing numbers of plates spinning on sticks. I had survived the neonatal ICU with the considerable support of Doctor Strickland and some wonderful nurses. I felt fortunate to have suffered only the Baby Boy Selness mishap and had learned much about the care of premature infants from the rotation. I hoped future rotations would be less eventful and imagined them to be less stressful. My assumptions would, of course, prove to be wrong.

**August 10**

Not many weeks later, I found myself assigned to the service where I had wished to begin my internship, the internal medicine service. I felt much more comfortable examining and treating adult patients than I had when dealing with preemies.

Once or twice a month during my internship I rode the night ambulance at the Old General to make extra money. We would respond to emergency calls such as strokes, overdoses, and heart attacks. A regularly scheduled stop was at the Minneapolis City Jail. Most requests there amounted to thinly veiled ruses to gain tranquilizers and narcotic medicines. I felt compassion for the incarcerated. Many of the prisoners were frightened and sought medicinal mental numbing. But my principles prevented me from giving in to their drug-seeking ways.

One evening we were scheduled to enter a neighborhood on the near north side in which an intern had earlier been assaulted by drug seekers. For my protection, a security guard from the hospital, complete with sidearm, rode along that evening. We encountered no difficulty at our stops, although once while hauling a medicine bag full of narcotics up four dark flights of stairs in a seedy tenement building, I admit to having felt unnerved. The dark corners and ominous shadows hastened the pace of my steps.

While riding the night away in the ambulance, Jack Barnett, the security officer, and I passed the time in desultory conversation. I noticed his surprise when I mentioned having admitted Alfonse D'Amico, a courtly eighty-three-year-old man, that afternoon.

The purpose for mentioning the patient was Mr. D'Amico's strong choice of the General for his health care. His financial security would have allowed him to obtain his care at fancier, private hospitals in the Twin Cities, many of which offered private beds, better food, and more individualized services. Alternatively, he could have traveled sixty miles south to Rochester and the famous Mayo Clinic. Now that was a place that knew how to market its health care. Mr. D'Amico, however, had unflinching loyalty to the General and told me he would never consider any hospital other than the Hennepin County General Hospital.

"So he's your patient, is he?" Jack said, nervously strumming his thin fingers on the well-secured litter. I noticed that Jack had a funny tic-like facial grimace.

"Sure is. Nice old gentleman."

"Watch yourself," Jack said in his clipped New York accent. I saw his face again twitch into a grimace.

"You know him?" I asked.

"Nah, know his son, Joey." Jack tugged at the collar of his uniform shirt.

"So?" I said.

"You don't know?" he said. In the interior lighting of the ambulance, I saw his dark eyebrows arch to a peak.

"Never heard of him."

"Not from around here, are you, doc?" His tone sounded condescending. "Joey's on TV, in the papers a lot, head of a big union. Law enforcement knows him, shall we say, for other reasons. You see, Joey's connected to the rackets—got quite a reputation too." There it was again, the pursing of his mouth into a grimace.

Jack had been a police officer in Minneapolis for many years before transferring to the slower-paced hospital security service. But despite a several-year interval, Jack's memory of police matters in the Twin Cities went as deep as a hooker's cleavage. After hearing a number of his stories, I began to wonder if his past work had jaded Jack's view of life.

"Wow, no pressure here. Can't wait for the family conference when we talk about dear old Dad," I said. "You think I'll need a security escort," I added, only half jokingly. Jack Barnett did not respond, but peered at me knowingly with his dark eyes and again made that funny facial grimace.

## August 11

As I drove from south Minneapolis into work the following morning, Jack's warning created a tickle of apprehension deep within the gray matter. Later while on work rounds, I spotted a well-dressed younger man at Mr. D'Amico's bedside with a striking resemblance to my patient. Sure enough he introduced himself as Joey D'Amico, but he failed to fit the image I had conjured up of him. The younger Mr. D'Amico wore an impeccably tailored dark pinstriped suit, red silk tie, and fancy imported shoes. He had wavy black hair and an olive complexion, and he spoke forcefully yet politely. He appeared to be well educated and listened attentively to everything I said.

"So how's Dad doing?" he began.

"He is doing well. We found an area of consolidation—that is, pneumonia in his right lung base—and have started intravenous antibiotics. He will be receiving pulmonary therapy twice a day. He is on oxygen now but mainly as a precaution." The strong smell of the younger Mr. D'Amico's flowery aftershave wafted over me as I spoke. The scent was unknown to me but smelled both manly and exotic.

"Any idea how long he'll be in the hospital?" Joey asked. He sat in a bedside chair, standing out from other less well-dressed visitors on the men's ward.

"Likely seven to ten days; depends on how fast the infection responds to our treatment."

Joey nodded his head, appearing satisfied with my answers.

In fact, the pneumonia on X-ray later proved slow to clear. Since the advent of Diagnosis-Related Groups (DRG) in the 1980s, specified time frames for any particular diagnosis are spelled out, with reimbursement for the ordained time to treat the illness. In this pre–DRG era, however, I was allowed more than two weeks to observe the interaction between father and son.

The senior Mr. D'Amico enjoyed daily visits and intermittent phone calls from his son. He would brighten considerably on Joey's arrival and always gave his son a big bear hug upon departure. Joey often brought his dad personal items such as newspapers, razor blades, and changes of pajamas and bathrobes. He also brought fruit and expensive chocolates for his dad and gave similar gifts to the nurses and me. He was solicitous and loving toward his father and would read the *Minneapolis Star and Tribune* to his low-vision father. Father and son often talked about sports and local politics. Beyond that, Joey could not have been more polite or respectful in his interaction with the nurses and me. He was certainly a big shot in town, but he did not act like one.

Years later I would see mention in the paper or on television of Joey D'Amico. The articles and reports would prompt my recall of his unflagging support for his father and how he had become the darling of the nurses. I never ran into a more solicitous family member. My own impression, based on my limited experience with Joey, differed from Jack's stark and unyielding opinion.

Admittedly I was pleased and relieved when the senior Mr. D'Amico was healthy enough to be discharged. I never knew nor wished to know what consequences might befall me if the senior Mr. D'Amico had taken a turn for the worse or if I had seriously screwed up his care. The presence of supportive and inquisitive family members in the hospital makes a big difference, especially when they are senior Mafia types.

After a challenging beginning, my intern year smoothed out and I steadily gained at least a modicum of self-confidence. The benefit of my rotating internship was it provided an opportunity to sample medicine from different specialty areas. I already had my residency lined up at the University of Minnesota in neurology and chose my elective rotations in areas I hoped would prove useful. These included ophthalmology, neurosurgery, and ear, nose, and throat.

My intern's wage was livable, barely. Trudy and I had rented the first floor of what was referred to in Minneapolis as a double bungalow, or duplex, on Twenty-ninth Avenue South. The owner's mother lived on the second floor. Because she did not own a car, she allowed us the use of the detached garage—valuable during the snowy Minnesota winters. In addition, the garage offered a place to plug in the engine-warming device. Now that was helpful on frigid mornings!

Trudy and I ate a lot of tuna and noodle casserole that year, short on the tuna. On rare occasion, we would motor downtown to Café Di Napoli, our favorite Italian restaurant on Hennepin, for meatballs and spaghetti. We would, if the finances allowed, spring for a bottle of inexpensive Chianti. The restaurant had whitewashed brick walls and red-and-white-checked tablecloths. Wine bottles adorned the tables with their multicolored wavelets of candle drippings.

Trudy's pregnancy caused her to develop the appetite of a barracuda. I recall the joy in her twinkling blue eyes when the large plate of pasta descended before her. Watching her delight, I felt personal affirmation for at last being the breadwinner for our small but growing family.

Interns received three full meals a day and ample leftovers at the midnight meal. On occasion I sneaked food home for Trudy or else invited her to join me in the hospital's cafeteria. The hospital was benevolent to its house staff in this and many other ways. For example, interns had reasonably quiet call rooms if we could ever break away from our hospital duties. And there was one unusual work benefit for house staff: free obstetrical care. This would prove extremely beneficial for Trudy and me.

**March 19, 1973**

I reported to work on obstetrics that morning, my mind gauzy with worry and sleep deprivation. Trudy was three weeks overdue with our first child with the weather report promising a blizzard. The ominous sky that morning had been leaden with gray, threatening clouds.

*Hold on, Trudy. Please don't go into labor today.*

My mother had flown in from Dallas earlier, wishing to be present for the birth and fearing I would be on call when Trudy's time came. Mom's instincts were once again right on.

I knew my mother had never driven in a Minnesota blizzard, nor had she ever negotiated any serious winter weather. But if Trudy went into labor while I was bottled up at the hospital, I knew my plucky mother would do everything possible to transport my young wife to the hospital.

The nineteenth of March proved busy, mercifully providing distraction from my personal worries. I made patient rounds, delivered six babies, performed multiple circumcisions, and carried out five newborn examinations. Around 3:00 a.m. on the twentieth, I heard the jolting words I most dreaded.

"Doctor Hutton, your wife is on the phone," said Gretchen. The obstetrics nurse called the disturbing message through a cracked door into the delivery room where I sat on a stool beneath a woman who was in the stirrups—and pushing.

The significance of Trudy's call struck me with all the force of an eighteen-wheeler. Unfortunately, I verged on delivering a baby who had just then begun to crown. I was torn between the utter necessity of delivering that baby and the enormous emotional draw to sprint for the telephone.

"Gretchen, I'll call as soon as I deliver this baby. Please find out what's going on."

*As if I don't already know.*

Not long after, I suctioned the new baby's nostrils and mouth, hurriedly clamped and severed the umbilical cord, handed off a crying, healthy neonate to the nurse in attendance, and delivered and inspected the placenta. I then streaked out of the delivery room, ripping off gloves and gown, and speed-dialed Trudy.

"My water broke," Trudy said with a faint tremor in her

voice. My mind immediately recalled television reports describing the city as utterly paralyzed by whiteout conditions.

"It's going to be fine, honey," I lied. "We've got it all covered. Can you please put Mom on the phone?" A moment later my mother was on the line. "Mom, think you can drive through the snowstorm to the hospital?" We had practiced the route days before, anticipating just such an emergency. "I'm sorry, our ambulances aren't running, so that option is out."

"Then I have to. Trudy is having contractions," Mom said, her voice faint but determined.

Human determination achieved landing men on the moon, digging the Panama Canal, and trekking to the far poles of the earth. With this same resolve, Mom miraculously managed to maneuver through snow-clogged streets during one of the most dreadful spring blizzards in Minnesota history. Minnesotans, sensible people that they are, stayed safely inside. Meanwhile, the determined mother-in-law from the sunny south with Trudy moaning softly in the backseat plowed through their snow-covered streets.

After what seemed like hours, I met Trudy and my mother in the emergency room. Mom looked as pale as overly bleached cotton. As the intern on call, I was responsible for all obstetrical admissions, even that of my own wife.

*This is just not right. A doctor is not supposed to treat his own family.*

I examined and confirmed that Trudy was in active labor. I tried unsuccessfully to calm my mother, who by then had realized the magnitude of her risky accomplishment. I found her blithering on to a glassy-eyed drunk in the waiting room about her frantic trek to the hospital. He nodded periodically in response, no doubt hoping this semihysterical woman might slip him a ten spot for a bottle. Seeing what was going on, I retrieved Mom and took her back into Trudy's cubicle.

I drew blood work from Trudy, completed her paperwork, slipped my mother a Valium, and rolled Trudy's gurney off to labor and delivery.

I tried to summon the obstetrical chief resident who had agreed to deliver Trudy, but this proved unsuccessful. Fred Kravitz told me that despite great effort he could not escape his snow-clogged driveway. It simply was too steep.

"Come on, Fred, Mom made it through snow-obstructed streets in the same snowstorm, and for goodness' sakes, she's from Texas!" My attempt at shaming this proud denizen of the northlands was fruitless.

"Tom, I tried and just can't make it. Have a long uphill driveway. The snow is ass deep to a moose," said Fred. "Really sorry, you'll just have to deliver Trudy yourself."

*Jesus Christ, this is the baby I'll drop, I just know it.*

Between my training at Baylor med and my internship at the General, I had delivered nearly two hundred babies. While versed in the mechanics of birthing, I worried what would happen if a complication arose.

An hour later I rechecked the status of Trudy's labor. She had not dilated further. This was odd, because she had been in active labor. Gretchen, whom I had known and trusted in the NICU, suggested we place a monitoring device on the baby. *Thank goodness Gretchen has a clear head.* We rigged the equipment and recorded the baby's heart rate along with Trudy's regular and forceful contractions.

Another two hours passed with Trudy laboring hard the whole time. She had earlier dilated to five centimeters, but beyond that Trudy's cervix would not go. Her cervix proved as stubborn as belly fat.

An urgent phone query to the snowbound chief resident resulted in my ordering pelvic X-rays. I soon received a dispiriting call from the radiologist, describing a critical narrowing of Trudy's midpelvis. This constriction prevented the baby's head from passing any farther down the birth canal. In short, the baby had his head stuck in a too small pipe. He was in imminent danger and required an immediate caesarean section.

I had never witnessed a caesarean, much less performed one. I needed an obstetrician like a fish needs water, yet in response to my worries, the blizzard outside only intensified. My desperate thoughts were firing off like kernels in a popper when Gretchen at Trudy's bedside loudly shouted for me.

"Doctor Hutton, look at this," she said. I hurried over and scanned the printout. The monitoring demonstrated a substantial drop in the baby's heart rate during a hard contraction. The heart rate of the baby slowed to a frightening rate, indicating the baby was in substantial distress. I tried not to show my alarm in front of Trudy but doubt I was successful.

I scampered for a telephone, called the ambulance shed, and spoke (yelled?) to the attendant, Glen. I begged him to retrieve the marooned chief obstetrics resident from his suburban home.

"Ambulances can't run tonight. Snow's too high, visibility next to nothing." I heard Glen making slurping sounds.

Nonplussed, I explained the situation and its gravity. I pled my case with all the urgency a desperate husband and imminent father could muster.

The slurping sound stopped. I sensed Glen, whom I knew to be a father, weakening. "Well, I'll try. Now doggone it, probably end up stuck or dead in a snowbank, but gosh darn it, I'll give it a shot."

"God bless you," I said. I hung up the telephone and contemplated the sorry situation.

It was only then that the possibility of a disastrous outcome fully dawned on me, a result I felt helpless to prevent. At that moment, I ceased thinking like a doctor and embraced my role as husband and father. Fear, worry, and anxiety crashed down upon me like a tsunami. I felt a sob building in my chest. I stood and retreated into an empty, darkened delivery room. There the dam of my reserve gave way.

Gretchen must have witnessed my senseless retreat because soon, on crepe soles, she silently entered. I felt consoling arms wrap around a sobbing me. She murmured that the ambulance would get through, that Glen was a skillful driver, and that the lives of my baby and wife would be saved. I desperately wanted to believe her. I had never been so frightened in my entire life.

It is far different treating members of your own family. The usual professional distance is lost. Objectivity becomes impossible. I reacted as a potential father and husband, not as the physician who at the time was in charge of obstetrics. The old medical aphorism came to mind: a doctor who treats himself or his family most assuredly has a fool for a patient. Yet under these circumstances, what choice did I have?

I stared, transfixed by the printouts, as I sat by Trudy's bedside. Time passed with all the rapidity of an aged sloth.

Amazingly and against all odds, within an hour and a half Fred Kravitz bounced out of the stairwell and into the obstetrical ward, grinning like a kid at a carnival. In his wake Glen followed, a smile on his face as big as Lake Superior. Using chains and determination, Glen had plucked Fred from his snowbound home and transported him to the hospital. I felt like planting big wet smackers on both of them.

Fred reviewed the monitoring strips, called the operating room for an emergency caesarean, and firmly slapped me on the back.

"Buck up! You're about to become a dad. We'll get your baby out before you can finish reciting the cranial nerves. Trudy and the baby will be fine. Want to go in the operating room and assist?"

Normally I would have jumped at the opportunity, but declined to observe my wife's bulging belly slit open like a gutted deer. I waited within the operating room suite but out of view of the procedure.

True to Fred's word, a nurse soon presented me a baby swaddled in warm blanket and with a great set of lungs.

"Doctor Hutton, meet your son."

My relief was palpable. Despite being exhausted, having not slept in more than twenty-four hours, I felt exhilarated like few times in my life. The nurse assured me that Trudy was fine but needed more suturing. I practically skipped out of the operating suite and carried Andy off to the newborn nursery. There I performed his newborn examination. To me, he looked absolutely perfect.

*No bias here.*

The running joke for several days was Hutton was the easiest intern in the hospital to locate. It was said I no longer needed paging, as I could be found either in the newborn nursery playing with my son, Andy, or at Trudy's bedside.

Trudy came through the caesarean without incident. She was a remarkable and courageous trooper. Fred discharged her early, saying I could care for her as well at home as I could at the hospital and she would be more comfortable at home.

I left the obstetrical service not owing a thin dime to the hospital—great intern benefit that was. Even more important, I left with a life-changing bonus, our first child. Not every intern had such luck, but admittedly I felt that I had worked my butt off to earn the soft bundle in my arms.

In the car on the way home, Trudy and I beamed goofily at each other. My mother rode in the backseat, having by then recovered from her middle-of-the-night heroic charge to the hospital. Andy, buried within a tiny red parka, cooed from Trudy's lap. Trudy and I could not have been prouder.

*Chapter 5*

# SLEUTHING AT THE VA

*We must choose between reality and madness.*

—Billy Joel

"Mr. Barnett, is someone trying to murder you?" I posed this highly unusual question to a man with a sullen expression and a pencil-thin mustache. His laserlike gaze bored into me for an uncomfortable period of time before he responded.

"Sonny, you're the damned doctor," he sneered from his hospital bed. "You figure it out!"

Two weeks previously, I could never have imagined engaging in such a provocative interview. I had just become the new neurology chief resident at the one-thousand-bed Minneapolis VA Medical Center. Earlier that morning I had left Building 2, which housed its neurological wards, and strode down a long corridor, connecting to a series of outbuildings. The extended passageway curved like the tail of a giant scorpion. I was responding to a recent consultation request.

As I made my way down the hallway, I periodically observed walkways leading off to side annexes. Each successive building seemed to house a still-longer-hospitalized group of veterans. When I gazed out the corridor's windows, I saw trees just beginning to leaf out. It was late afternoon during the spring of 1976. The faint echo of my footsteps and the clinking of medical instruments within my black bag gave a cavernous, lonely sound to my solitary hike. I had never before ventured to these deep recesses of the hospital. I certainly never expected to encounter the most bizarre case of my life, indeed to come across the black swan of my medical career.

After a brisk ten-minute walk to the end of the hallway, I reached Building 7, the rehabilitation ward, and the location of the most chronic of the hospital's patients. Most had resided on the rehabilitation ward for months, if not years. Local lore claimed some veterans had arrived with the hospital's opening in 1925 and had never left.

*If the Minneapolis VAMC is an acute VA hospital, what then do the chronic VA hospitals look like? Good grief, what about the VA domiciliaries?*

The consult request read: "57-year-old, service-connected veteran with numbness and tingling of feet and legs." Usually this pedestrian complaint, especially from a chronic ward, predicted an unexciting and unrewarding consult for peripheral neuropathy. Such an assumption could not have been further from the truth.

"I came here to recuperate three months ago, after three weeks in the intensive care unit, several more on the medical ward," said Robert Barnett.

*He must qualify as a veritable newcomer on this ward.*

Barnett had penetrating dark eyes and a slight build. *Curmudgeon* came to mind. But by far his most remarkable characteristic was his expressive voice. It was deep in tone with a slow, tailing-off, vibrating quality, like the voice of Henry Kissinger. Barnett's descending and prolonged voice sizzle projected absolute authority and unquestioned self-confidence.

"The numbness, burning, and tingling came later, and got worse. Can't walk," he said in his rich, resounding voice. His speech demonstrated little emotion other than subtle inflections.

From reviewing his chart, I learned that on entering the hospital he had been profoundly ill with severe diarrhea, vomiting, belly pain, and suppression of his bone marrow. For the first several weeks, Barnett's very survival had been in question. He required massive amounts of intravenous fluids, repeated blood transfusions, and tube feedings. Laboratory tests revealed mild liver and kidney problems as well. Despite a raft of tests and a cadre of medical specialists, no specific cause for his illness had ever been determined.

He later developed a curious rash that eventually became scaly. Again no clear reason for this had been determined. Barnett eventually stabilized and was shipped off the acute medical service to recuperate in this, the final building in the arc of outbuildings.

"What type of work have you done?" I asked as I settled into the chair at his bedside.

"After discharge from the army, I taught college for several years, but no longer."

"Why did you leave that line of work?"

"Didn't work out." He shifted his gaze, indicating to me that line of questioning was at an end.

"What are you doing now?" I asked.

"Not much; don't teach anymore." Our conversation was briefly interrupted by an intercom announcement advertising an upcoming bake sale.

"How do you support yourself?"

"Service-connected VA pension."

"Are you doing part-time work or other activities?"

"Well, in a way, kind of a religious man, you might say."

Despite persisting with follow-up questions, I could gain little additional information on his religious activities or details about his departure from the teaching field. Strange, I thought. He doesn't share much.

*I wonder if he is guarded or suspicious?*

Robert did boast of his genius IQ, a finding later born out on psychological testing. His extensive vocabulary and breadth of knowledge provided tacit validity for his potential membership in Mensa.

*Learning his medical history will be slow going. How unusual for a man of his intellectual firepower to remain unemployed.*

My examination that day revealed atrophy of the muscles of his feet and hands and absent reflexes. Barnett also had reduced sensation below his knees to light touch and pinprick sensation and to a lesser degree a glovelike sensory loss in his hands. Although numb, his feet proved extremely painful when lightly touched.

*Numb yet painful. What an unfortunate combination, anesthesia dolorosa.*

When I moved his great toe out of his view, Barnett could not discern the position of the toe, or if it was even moving. His walking was unsteady.

*He has severe loss of proprioception out of proportion with his primary sensory loss.*

That he was suffering a severe peripheral neuropathy with some involvement of the spinal cord was clear. Barnett appeared, however, not to have the common causes for neuropathy, such as diabetes mellitus or alcoholism. He denied exposure to a long list of toxic substances, solvents, or vitamin deficiencies, and he had no medical condition that caused peripheral neuropathy.

*This is not going to be easy.*

I ordered a battery of tests, admittedly usually unrewarding ones, but on occasion revealing cryptic causes for peripheral neuropathy and spinal cord disease. Having initiated the neurological evaluation, I departed the rehab ward for the day.

A week later I again walked the long angling hallway to pay a follow-up visit on Barnett. I was pleased to learn a medicine I had prescribed had relieved the burning of his palms and soles. The test results that had returned to the chart, not surprisingly, were unrevealing. With little else to discuss, I inquired further about his home life.

"Married ten years but separated," he said.

"Where is your wife living?"

"Lives in the house; she lives on one floor, I live on another, share some things," he replied with his voice descending again into the tonal basement.

"That's an unusual arrangement," I said, attempting to draw him out.

"Cheaper that way. It works," he said. His coal black eyes bore into me and made me feel uncomfortable.

"Are you leading separate lives?"

"She cooks for us, and I help her out some. We share a few things." Strange, I thought, how each of his answers leaves something dangling. Mildly maddening even, I thought. The whole time, he scrutinized me with his searing eyes and hostile expression. Following my questions, his speech had deliberate pauses during which he carefully constructed his answers. The way he gamed me with his responses made me wonder if he was playing an intellectual cat-and-mouse game with me.

The following week, as I sat in my office, I received an urgent telephone call from the chemistry laboratory. An excited lab technician informed me Robert Barnett's urine arsenic value was extremely elevated—the highest he had ever seen. He asked if I knew the source of his intoxication.

"Haven't a clue," I responded. In truth, I had ordered the battery of tests for completeness, not having been particularly suspicious of arsenic intoxication. But immediately on learning the result, I realized the elevated arsenic level precisely explained the initial abdominal complaints, skin changes, reduced blood count and platelets, as well as the delayed onset of peripheral neuropathy. Later examination of Barnett's nails confirmed classic Mees' lines—linear white streaks in fingernails and toenails—consisting of deposited arsenic. Determining the rate of nail growth and measuring the distance of the line from its origin would precisely date the intoxication.

I soon visited Barnett and informed him of the abnormal arsenic result. He looked at me quizzically but said nothing. I posed questions on potential sources of arsenic intoxication, but my queries proved unrewarding. Barnett urged me, even challenged me to find the source of his poisoning.

I knew a common cause for arsenic poisoning was attempted homicide. On my third visit, I asked the obvious but most challenging question that began this story.

"Nope, don't know anyone who wants me dead."

"Do you have a lot of life insurance?" I asked. This question resulted in a rare but limited show of emotion, consisting of a chuckle and a shaking of his head.

"Well, if you don't mind me asking, how is your relationship with your estranged wife?"

"Matilda? I don't think she's got it in her. Don't get along all that well, but can't see her trying to finish me off. Still . . ."

He had done it again, trailing off on a question before answering it. He again declined to elaborate.

Further questions revealed a neighbor who spent an unusual amount of time in the house. Bruce, the male friend, and Matilda were frequently together in her portion of the house. What Bruce and Matilda did there, Barnett seemed not to have a clue. It was also apparent that a veritable troop of young, principally female college-age students frequented Barnett's portion of the house but for reasons that remained unclear to me.

Why? Questions as to their purpose in the house were evaded. Maddening.

As I departed the chronic rehabilitation ward that day, I observed four women in their midtwenties with long, straight hair, heading toward Barnett's bed. They had a languid bearing about them.

I wonder why they're here?

On Wednesday of the following week, I met with Barnett's estranged wife in a private conference room in the chronic rehabilitation building. Matilda was in her midsixties, of short stature, with pulled-back gray hair and no makeup. She was plain-looking and hardly fit my gestalt of a murderess. In contrast to the forceful speech of her estranged husband, Matilda spoke meekly. Most of the interview was unrevealing, but once she briefly let her veil of caution drop.

"Robert mentioned you have a friend by the name of Bruce who spends a lot of time in your home," I probed.

"Ridiculous he would even mention Bruce after the trollops who visit him," she said with a sneer. I saw her posture stiffen and her jaw tighten.

"Are you suspicious of the women?" I asked.

"More suspicious of that old lecher," Matilda spat out. She seemed uncomfortable with having shared this piece of information and declined to say anything more on the subject.

When later the two of us visited Robert's bedside, she changed her demeanor quicker than a chameleon changes its color. She acted subservient to Robert. I observed him repeatedly cut her off midsentence. I also observed Matilda visibly cringe in response to his periodic admonishments.

*Such abusive treatment leads to resentment. Could it provoke Matilda to stronger actions still?*

The medical question of whether to treat his arsenic intoxication perplexed me. The medical literature of the day was vague about whether leeching the body of arsenic after this time delay would help. I ordered a course of chelation just to be safe. Urine values of arsenic immediately spiked with the treatment, showing at least the effectiveness of the therapy at mobilizing arsenic out of his body.

After careful consideration and checking with hospital administration, I decided to report the arsenic intoxication to the Minneapolis police, suggesting Barnett might represent an attempted homicide. A bored officer received my telephone report and said he would look into the matter.

As it was my first time to make a diagnosis of arsenic intoxication, I felt a degree of accomplishment. But I remained frustrated by my inability to identify the source, souring any feelings of real fulfillment. Over the following weeks and months, Barnett showed improvement in his arm and leg strength and his ability to move about. His body weight increased. Eventually he was well enough to be discharged from the hospital. Could he be one of the rare ones to be discharged alive from what I had begun to think of as the hospital's Siberia?

•••

Time seemed to fly by, with me completing my residency training and then joining the faculty. In the fall of 1977, I again found myself breathing the astringent-scented air of the Minneapolis VAMC, but this time as a newly minted staff physician. I had climbed onto the first rung of the academic ladder, becoming an instructor at the University of Minnesota's Department of Neurology. This also provided me the opportunity to continue working on my PhD from the university.

Not long after my return to the VA, to my surprise I again encountered Robert Barnett. I was shocked to learn that in the interim he had been admitted several additional times for recurring bouts of arsenic poisoning. On those occasions, his illness had been less severe than his first and had been immediately suspected. He received additional courses of chelating agent and regularly improved. Repeat medical evaluations had again failed to reveal a reason or source for his arsenic intoxication.

"Mr. Barnett, you're getting to be a regular here," I said, extending my hand to shake. When I gripped his hand, I felt the muscular wasting of his hand consistent with his peripheral neuropathy. (Herein I offer a trade secret of neurologists. When they shake hands, they focus more on the distribution and quantity of the hand muscles than on mere social graces.)

"Seems that way," he said somberly. "Feet and hands acting up again. The burning and tingling came back, my walking and use of my fingers got worse. . . ." His sizzling voice trailed off.

"You sure you don't work with any chemicals, or have access to chemistry labs?"

"Nope," he responded in his avuncular fashion.

"No woodworking or access to treating wood?"

"No."

"Any exposure to insecticides or products to kill rodents?"

"Not that either."

"What about your relationship with your wife?"

He scrutinized me carefully before responding. "Same as always. Spends time with Bruce, the neighbor guy." In reviewing the history of his multiple bouts of arsenic intoxication, suspiciously Bruce had always been in the Barnetts' house just prior to Mr. Barnett falling ill.

"Do you know what Bruce does for a living?"

"Works for a chemical company."

*Bingo. Might Bruce have access to arsenic? Is this an awkward lover's triangle with Mr. Barnett representing an inconvenient third person?*

"How do you and Bruce get along?"

"Okay. My wife's friend, not mine."

The urine tests again revealed elevated levels of arsenic, but not as high as on Barnett's initial admission. A social worker and psychologist tried to gain a greater understanding of the curious home situation and get insights into Barnett's psyche. His marked defensiveness limited the information that could be obtained, but nevertheless, they heard hints of wrongdoing about his wife and Bruce. Robert also dropped vague intimations of possible sources of the arsenic and motivation for his poisoning, but no compelling substantiation existed that could determine malfeasance.

The Minneapolis Police Department interviewed the neighbor, the wife, and the patient as well. When I followed up with the officer, he could determine no clear involvement of Bruce that would stand up in court. He was even less certain regarding his opinion of Mrs. Barnett.

*Someone is slipping him arsenic, but who?*

I next called the Minneapolis Department of Health. I knew the Health Department had an epidemiologist on staff, and I sought his expertise. After I detailed the case and after much cajoling, he responded favorably. I sensed he was tired of chasing outbreaks of food-borne illnesses, stemming largely from Minneapolis's plethora of smorgasbords.

Despite unrevealing searches of the home by both Mr. and Mrs. Barnett, I asked their permission to look around the home. The couple granted my request and seemed, at least on the surface, anxious to find the source for the arsenic. The epidemiologist and I arranged for a time to meet at the Barnetts' home and carry out a further search.

The following agreed-upon Tuesday afternoon arrived. I departed the hospital driving my used Buick that formerly had belonged to National Car Rental. In its earlier life as a rental, it had been wrecked, fixed, and finally sold. It was not in the best condition, but the price had been affordable.

From the hospital, I took a quick jog over to Minnehaha Avenue and drove north on the busy road. I passed by Minnehaha Falls already crowded with tourists seeking the location made famous by Henry Wadsworth Longfellow in his epic poem *Hiawatha*. Ironically, Longfellow had never actually visited the falls but had merely read about them.

I eventually turned onto Hiawatha Avenue until reaching East Forty-sixth Street. I made a right turn and headed toward the Mississippi River. Before reaching the river, I turned left into a tree-lined residential area of stately old homes.

I met Doctor Max Levy, the epidemiologist, in front of a gray, old castle of a house. From the curbside, the three-story house looked austere, run down, dark, and vaguely ominous. Its size alone would make our search challenging.

I took a key from my pocket, provided me earlier, and entered the front hallway. I stood for a long moment, absorbing the environment. The first floor was furnished with old, heavy wooden furniture.

I soon located Mrs. Barnett's bedroom. I surmised this from finding women's clothing stuffed into a large closet. The next room we investigated was the kitchen. It had an old Chambers range and a still more senior Oldman's refrigerator with a condenser on top emitting heat. The metal box had a vintage fastener on the door. A small, round kitchen table with two red, vinyl-covered chairs fit cozily into the corner.

Between the kitchen and bedroom was a light and airy sewing room that had an impressive number of skeins of various-colored yarn. We searched every room on the first floor including all the drawers, cabinets, and cases. We found no arsenic or anything else of a suspicious nature.

We then climbed a tight, creaking stairway to the second floor. On arriving at the top, our attention was inexorably drawn to the unusual décor in one of its rooms. The area had originally been designed as a study with dark wooden panels but had been converted into a chapel of some sort. An altar stood at the far end of the room. Behind it appeared several vaguely familiar religious symbols. While some were Christian, the array appeared ecumenical, with Muslim, Buddhist, and Shinto symbols present also. Some I failed to recognize altogether. The floor bore thick, worn black carpeting. Various incense holders, a fat Buddha, and numerous candles adorned the tables. The tables held vases containing dried flowers and sprays of marijuana leaves. The tables flanked four stark wooden pews. The predominant colors in the room consisted of rich Titian reds and inky blacks. A rock fireplace occupied the far end of the room.

Just outside the chapel was an even smaller stairway that led to the attic and to an extraordinary room. There was enough room for two comfortable-appearing couches with side tables. Heavy red-velvet drapes obscured the light. Posters and figurines depicting various positions of the Kama Sutra decorated walls and tables. Several low-wattage lamps with red lightbulbs perched on tables. A large statue of Aphrodite held sway. On a cabinet, a high-fidelity record player resided with albums heavy on sitar music, medieval chants, and a few classics including Ravel's *Bolero*. Winged and tailed devils with pitchforks and whips adorned bookshelves. The room contained an eclectic collection of old and new erotica and a broad array of religious and occult symbols.

*All we need now is for Bela Lugosi to skulk out from a hidden door and cue a spooky soundtrack.*

Although what we saw was odd, none of it added up to attempted murder by poison. Over time we searched every floor including the basement. After three hours we despaired over not finding anything of value toward solving our case. Then, I discovered in a corner of the dank basement an out-of-the-way hiding place. Within an old sewing-machine case and hidden in a hatbox, I found a partial case of Terro Ant Killer. From my reading of the label, I learned the active ingredient was sodium arsenate. I yelled upstairs for Max and soon heard him noisily clomping down the stairway.

"Is this stuff legal?" I asked, holding up a bottle of Terro for his inspection.

"Terro and several other varieties of sodium arsenate–containing ant killers are on the market, perfectly legal, and easily obtainable," he replied.

"This is a lot of ant killer. Can't imagine that big a problem with ants," I said.

The accompanying information with the bottle said Terro Ant Killer contained sucrose—table sugar—and attracted sugar-eating ants that would take the lethal meal to the queen, eventually wiping out the entire colony. Max and I discussed the discovery excitedly. Both of us believed the sodium arsenate was the basis for Barnett's recurring arsenic intoxication.

"I've heard of Terro Ant Killer causing accidental arsenic poisoning in children," said Max.

Close by the sewing box, we located two dusty medical textbooks. On review, we found underlined sections on arsenic intoxication. The texts provided descriptions of symptoms produced by arsenic and a brief section on treatment.

Among other information described in one of the books was the mysterious case of Ambassador Clare Boothe Luce's arsenic poisoning. Luce was a well-known American playwright, editor, journalist, and congresswoman before she was appointed by President Eisenhower to serve as the American ambassador to Italy.

The Luce poisoning drama played out in the 1950s before a breathless, worldwide audience. Given her strong anticommunist stance while living in a country not long before defeated by the victorious Allies, speculation arose whether the American ambassador was poisoned in a political intrigue. Ultimately her deteriorating health required she leave her ambassadorial post and return to the United States for treatment.

The cause of her arsenic intoxication eventually was traced to arsenic-containing paint chips that fell from her fresco-decorated bedroom. She habitually had enjoyed working while sitting in her bed, sipping coffee or tea. Over many months, flakes of arsenic-containing paint had fallen into her breakfast drink. The article within the medical text triumphantly declared that at long last the Luce medical mystery had been solved without the involvement of political intrigue.

Max Levy and I buzzed with enthusiasm.

"We got it, we found the source," I burbled.

"Yes, but now we must determine how the ant killer got from the bottle into Mr. Barnett," said the always-methodical epidemiologist.

"You're right," I said. "Several persons had access. Mrs. Barnett does the cooking and could have repeatedly dosed Mr. Barnett's food or drink with Terro. She could then have hidden the poison in the sewing box. Am willing to bet the sewing box is hers.

"I sensed when I interviewed her that she held a thinly veiled animosity toward Robert. After all, you have to admit he isn't the most lovable guy around."

"What about Bruce, the neighbor?" asked Max. "He might know the location of the arsenic or could have even hidden it there. Bruce could well be the culprit, as he's always around when Mr. Barnett falls ill. His situation in the home is a little bit too cozy. Plus his relationship with Mrs. Barnett might be more than platonic, as the two of them claim. He has probably seen how Mr. Barnett treats the missus. Maybe he is out for revenge."

The following day I was back in the rehabilitation unit at Barnett's bedside. When confronted with our observations on the chapel, Mr. Barnett reluctantly stated, "I started a religion based on truth seeking and deepening of our spiritual understanding." He declined to characterize the nature of his religion, its rituals, or his beliefs further. Barnett claimed he had applied for and received tax-exempt status for his church from the state of Minnesota. This sanctioning by the state pleased him greatly, as demonstrated by his first-ever smile in my presence. The small congregation was growing, he said, and consisted of people in their twenties and thirties. I was not surprised when Barnett informed me that he served as high priest.

Later, from interviews of his young female visitors, we learned religious services included smoking marijuana and hashish, chanting, and praying to a pantheon of gods.

"If one god is good, then a lot must be even better," had replied a young lady with long, blond hair and a vacuous facial expression.

Robert, as high priest, led these smoky, mind-altering ceremonies. Following this service, the group would recess to the erotica-filled room on the third floor with its thick carpets and comfortable couches. There the members would celebrate the beauty of the human body and stretch their sensual insights through liberated, guilt-free sexual acts. Barnett was described as wearing an elaborate white-fur-lined maroon robe that he would discard after the service. Underneath he was nude. His mostly female acolytes dressed in black would then undress and expand their collective consciousness by depleting their sexual energies.

When learning of the rituals practiced in the upper room, Max Levy and I pondered what this might add to our formulation of Barnett's mysterious case. We speculated arsenic might be used in an as yet undetermined role in the religious rituals or ceremonies, a sort of religious homeopathy. Also, we wondered if Mrs. Barnett's jealousy over Robert's dalliances with younger women might implicate her. We speculated, as well, whether religious seekers drawn to this unorthodox sect would be more likely to poison an overbearing, offish chief priest. All these clues proved grist for the mill of conjecture but failed to provide a final answer to the mystery.

*And my taxes are indirectly supporting this so-called religion.*

The medical team and Minneapolis Department of Health

stepped up their efforts. Interviews were conducted. We improved our understanding of Barnett's psyche. The behavioral health consultants described him as highly narcissistic and possessed with the belief he could communicate with his deceased mother by way of automatic handwriting. He showed paranoid tendencies and believed he was being spied on through one-way mirrors and hidden microphones. The shrinks diagnosed Barnett as having a narrowly confined delusional system that for years had escaped detection because of his marked defensiveness.

Unfortunately, we had no way in which we could carry out such testing on Mrs. Barnett or Bruce. What might a similar inspection of their psyches reveal?

However, we gained little additional insight into potential motives. Mrs. Barnett and Bruce agreed to provide urine samples for arsenic determination. When their reports returned, I dialed Max Levy.

"The arsenic values for Matilda Barnett and her frequent visitor, Bruce, are both negative," I said.

"Damn," exclaimed Max Levy. "I was building a case for contamination of the water supply to the house."

"How do you figure that?"

"A few instances of arsenic poisoning exist from naturally occurring arsenic deposits in the ground," Max said. "Now where do we go?"

"Tells us something at least," I said.

"What's that?" asked Max, a dejected tone in his voice.

"Well, tells us that since Robert Barnett is the only one with arsenic in his system, he must have been fed it. Improves the chances of poisoning!" I concluded.

The partial case of Terro Ant Killer was removed from the home. While we felt our shoe leather epidemiology had identified the source of his intoxication, we were forced to admit that we had made no progress in determining how Barnett repeatedly contracted his illness. It felt like we had made a long run up for a very short jump.

During the summer of 1978, Barnett made his eighth appearance on the VA neurology inpatient ward. My ward team was not scheduled to take admissions that day, but my interest (some would call it obsession) had become well known. When I saw his name on the admission list, I could not resist the temptation.

Admittedly, I possess a degree of doggedness in my personality—just ask my family. Over the preceding months and years, I had gone so far as to ask friends and colleagues to ponder the case with me. What were we missing? Was there a clue overlooked in this medical mystery?

I had obtained the input of the Health Department, the local police, and every medical consultant who potentially could offer help. This unsolved case had proved an enigma despite great expenditure of time and energy. The case of Robert Barnett had become a clinical vacuum cleaner for both time and resources.

The Homicide Division of the Minneapolis Police Department had nothing further to add. One droll homicide officer told me, "Call us when you have a body to investigate." While I thought his approach medically absurd, I could press him no further.

The arsenic conundrum had preyed on my mind. I found myself dreaming about Robert Barnett, rereading old mysteries to sharpen my skills of deduction, and assiduously studying each new article in the medical literature on arsenic intoxication. I mulled over the many disparate facts and obsessed at length over what I had missed.

No way would I miss another attempt at solving this whodunit. The opportunity to delve back into the case for me was clinical catnip.

Barnett again had his usual arsenic symptoms, suggesting he had once again another load on board. Laboratory tests confirmed our clinical suspicions.

"Any idea how you are picking up the arsenic, Mr. Barnett?" I asked.

"Nope."

"Mrs. Barnett still doing the cooking?" I asked. Again the pregnant pauses prior to his calculated rejoinders.

"Yes, sonny, Matilda still cooks for us." His dark, steady eyes never left my face. His voice revealed little inflection other than the distinctive sizzle of his voice.

"Has Bruce been in the house recently?"

"Every day I hear him simpering around," Robert said, irritation never far from his voice.

"What does he do while he is there?"

"Walks around, visits Matilda, talk—hell, ask him!"

Robert occasionally showed brief flare-ups of temper. I paused for a few seconds for his emotions to cool before proceeding.

"Mr. Barnett, do you think either Matilda or Bruce want you dead?"

"Can't imagine why, lovable guy that I am." He gave a wry smirk.

"Do you have a lot of money or anything else of great value?"

"No. Well, I do own about ten acres on Minnetonka Lake. Belonged to my mother. The land is surrounded by expensive homes and while I haven't checked it out, is probably valuable."

*I imagine it is valuable. That location is golden.*

"Any use of chemicals, particularly arsenic, in your rituals at your church?"

"No, not unless you count tetrahydrocannabinol."

"What do your services consist of?"

"Partake of a little pot, pray, sing, meditate, and celebrate the vast, liberating powers of tantric sexuality."

Barnett was unusually informative in this regard but otherwise proved less than forthcoming with our investigation. Like a stripper he would tantalize me with some flashed snippet, only to later withdraw it or minimize its significance. I felt that Barnett was tugging at the forelock of the medical profession and at me in particular. Hours of questioning, searches of his house, and multiple medical, epidemiological, and police investigations had failed to confirm motive or mechanism for his arsenic intoxication. To say that I was frustrated was akin to claiming the Irish like Guinness. I resolved once and for all to get to the bottom of the puzzle, no matter what it took.

After much consideration, I hatched an idea, really a long shot, but a previously untried approach. I would have to wait till the following week to put my thoughts into action.

In those days an advantage in the VA system was money for outside consultants. One consultant hired by the neurology service was an experienced psychiatrist, a Doctor Edmund Greenspan. I enjoyed his visits to our wards both because of his helpful service for our patients and for his courtly, Old World manner.

"Edmund, I heard you say once that you did sodium amytal interviews," I began one afternoon at the conclusion of his clinical teaching conference. I knew if I proved unsuccessful at this early stage, my idea would go no further.

"Yes, Tom, been known on occasion to use what some have called truth serum. I find on occasion that it expedites our typically laborious psychiatric process."

I shared the defensiveness of Robert Barnett that had befuddled us and also the mystery surrounding his repeated arsenic poisoning before asking, "You think a sodium amytal interview might break through his defensiveness and obtain straight answers for a change?"

I had been considering this approach for several weeks and knew at the very least it was unconventional. My persistence grew from a sense of desperation. I gazed upon the neatly dressed, elderly physician with his Sigmund Freud–like beard. I realized I was holding my breath.

Doctor Greenspan rubbed his chin and paused. "Might, just might," Edmund said, gazing thoughtfully off into the distance.

"Would you be willing to try it?" I asked, exhaling loudly.

Edmund looked at me with his gentle brown eyes, thought a moment, and responded, "Absolutely. Let's try it next week.

You order the tubing, syringes, and medicine, and we will interview your reticent Mr. Barnett."

My spirits soared. Suddenly I had a new direction and renewed hope. Perhaps this method would allow us to understand the hidden factors facing us.

By the following Tuesday, all was set. If Mr. Barnett's defensiveness were ever to be broken down, it would be on that day. Otherwise, our continued investigations would have as little hope for solving the mystery as would a pop bottle rocket hitting the moon.

The days for me had crawled by like a caterpillar with sore feet. But at last Tuesday afternoon arrived and found me on the second floor in a building attached by a hallway to the neurology floor. Nearby an intravenous kit rested on a metal tray. The short tubing had a receptacle through which the amytal would be injected. The medicine was equally divided between two syringes and lay on the gray metal tray.

The interview room was located in a quiet part of the hospital, a room frequently used by Doctor Greenspan for his psychiatric consultations. Shades covered the windows and a comfortable couch had been specially placed. The room was quiet, had low ambient lighting, and, I thought, had a surprisingly homey atmosphere for a federal building.

Doctor Greenspan, knowing of my great interest, had invited me to observe the interview. A comfortable, cushioned chair was placed in a corner of the room within easy hearing distance but removed from Mr. Barnett's line of sight.

The patient was scheduled to arrive at 1:15 p.m. By 1:30 he had not arrived, and I felt myself becoming restless. I realized time at the VAMC must be recorded differently than elsewhere in the world, but still. Finally, at 1:45 I heard an unhurried knock at the door. On opening the door the transportation service employee, without so much as a word of explanation, directed Barnett into the room and then turned to depart.

I shook Mr. Barnett's hand. "Thanks for your willingness to undergo an amytal interview," I said.

"Always glad to expand medicine's meager base of knowledge and personally gain new experiences," Mr. Barnett replied haughtily.

Doctor Greenspan oriented Barnett to the upcoming procedure. Greenspan led him to the couch and asked him to assume a comfortable position. With little ado, I slipped the needle into a vein on the back of Barnett's hand and taped the intravenous securely. I plugged in a bottle of saline fluid to clear the line and then retired to my observation post.

Doctor Greenspan began with relaxation exercises. He had Barnett begin deep breathing with slow exhalation. He went on by asking Barnett to relax his muscles beginning at the toes and slowly working upward through his body to his head. The soporific effect of Doctor Greenspan's voice was great, and I felt myself relaxing as well.

Doctor Greenspan tried briefly to interview Mr. Barnett without benefit of the sodium amytal but encountered Barnett's habitual defensiveness. He inserted the first syringe containing the sodium amytal into the rubber end of the tubing.

"You may begin to feel drowsy and relaxed. Just give into it, Robert," murmured the psychiatrist, as he began slowly injecting the liquid. Shortly thereafter Barnett began to speak in slower, less clipped sentences.

Edmund asked a series of historical questions. Barnett at first claimed a medical condition required him to stop teaching but eventually described his poor work performance at the college. We learned he had been asked to resign his teaching post. Robert said he had rankled under the authority of the college, and in an apparent show of obstinacy had been slow to post grades and submit the required paperwork.

*Hey, this seems to be working.* I felt hopeful.

"Where did you live when you returned to Minneapolis?" asked Doctor Greenspan.

"With Mama. The house I live in now belonged to her. She fixed my meals, washed my clothes, and provided money if I needed it," said Robert.

"Sounds like you had a good situation," said Doctor Greenspan.

"Wonderful, really, no worries at all. That is until Mama suddenly up and died." Barnett said this sounding more irritated than saddened.

"What did you do then?" asked Doctor Greenspan in his gentle voice.

"Mama's best friend Matilda kept coming to the house even after Mama's death and began cooking and cleaning; realized I couldn't do either. Eventually we just decided to marry so she wouldn't have to come and go every day. Proved convenient until we had a falling out," Barnett said.

"What was the falling out over?"

"Matilda didn't think much of my church."

"Robert, tell me where the arsenic ant killer came from?" asked Doctor Greenspan.

"Shop on Lake Street. Bought it and brought it home."

"Robert, why did you do that? Did you have an ant problem?"

"No, no ant problem."

"Well, why then, Robert?"

I felt my heart begin to race. I knew the moment of truth had arrived. Here we would either break through his defenses or we would not. I saw Doctor Greenspan inject a little more sodium amytal and switch to the second syringe. Robert seemed to relax even more, sagging into the couch. His breathing was deep and slow.

"I needed it for my condition," said Robert finally, his voice resonant and relaxed.

"What do you mean your condition, Robert?"

"When I was teaching, I got in a bad way. I lacked patience. I felt accountable for my job and didn't want the responsibility. I felt people were against me, spying on me. I didn't want anymore of that hard life."

"What did you do?"

"I began to think how I could make my life less stressful, began reading about medical conditions. Being disabled sounded like a great life. I was already receiving a VA pension, just needed to get it increased. I learned arsenic poisoning was difficult to diagnose and caused invalidism. Read how it interacted with proteins in the body and gave rise to an unusual array of symptoms. Got a hold of some arsenic at the college. Needed a way to retire without looking bad in Mama's eyes. I really wanted to go home to Mama." He said this with several muffled sobs.

"You mean you began to take arsenic?"

"Just before going back to Minneapolis, so Mama would feel sorry for me and let me stay with her."

"Tell me more about other times you used arsenic."

"Next time was 1977, when the VA called me in to reevaluate my service-connected disability. The doctor, a dumb intern, told me to go back to work, said my condition wasn't bad enough for disability. The son of a bitch! Couldn't sleep for days, fretting over that idiot's opinion. Figured his report would cancel my government checks!"

"What did you do next?"

The gentle yet persistent questioning of Edmund Greenspan impressed me. He was skillfully exploring the rugged terrain of Robert's suppressed memories.

"Came across Terro Ant Killer," said Robert. "Bought a case of it. Mixed up some and tried to kill myself. Couldn't face teaching again, didn't have any money. Mama had died. Fallen out with Matilda by then; life like that, I figured, was not worth living."

"Is that when you were first admitted and met Doctor Hutton?" Doctor Greenspan said, nodding in my direction.

"Hadn't figured the VA would pull me through or be smart enough to figure what was wrong with me. But as I lay in the rehab bed, I developed a plan. Could tell that I was improving, but I didn't want to improve enough some wiseass doctor would snatch away my disability check."

"So what did you do to prevent this, Robert?"

"Well, when I started to get better, I'd dose myself again. Had a pretty good idea by then how much Terro Ant Killer it would take for the right effect."

"How did you take the ant poison?"

"Tried different ways but found mixing it with beer was best. Especially liked it mixed with Leinenkugel."

"Why was that?"

"Killed the bitter taste."

"Robert, are you liable to take more arsenic in the future?"

"Would if my condition was threatened again. I've got it pretty good now."

I slumped back in my chair incredulous over the interview. The sodium amytal had proved successful beyond my greatest expectations. It revealed Barnett had been self-administering arsenic to maintain a state of chronic invalidism in order to avoid a world he perceived as overly demanding and threatening. Within his focused psychosis, his actions seemed altogether reasonable.

Later the question arose as to why Barnett had agreed to undergo a sodium amytal interview. While he never directly answered this question, it is my belief his arrogance and impressive intelligence overcame his better judgment. Basically, he was cocky and thought he could outsmart everyone else.

One last medical question required answering, and that was how to deal with this "frequent flier." Although we now understood his self-administration of arsenic, he professed a willingness to use it again. This presented a final and daunting challenge for our discharge planning of this patient.

Days later and after careful consideration, I offered Barnett an option for his living circumstances. This was based on having accessed his old military records. We discovered his service-connected disability had been for a psychiatric condition. My alternative provided regular meals, free and safe housing, and a place where his self-administration of arsenic could be avoided.

As it turned out, this option delighted Robert. Upon his discharge from the Minneapolis VAMC, Robert Barnett was transferred to a nearby chronic VA facility. To the best of my knowledge, he lived out the remainder of his life there, securely within the embrace of that VA facility. The system, after all, is not affectionately referred to as "Mother VA" for nothing.

In his new location, I later heard, Barnett received frequent visits from starry-eyed young ladies wearing long, straight hair and casual dress. From his private room, strange chants, smells, and sounds were often said to emanate.

*Free room and board, a VA pension, new intellectual sparring partners, and promiscuous acolytes—maybe Robert Barnett really does have life figured out.*

**Addendum**

My experience with Mr. Barnett and his Terro Ant Killer–related arsenic intoxication prompted me to survey twenty cases collected over a four-year period by the Minnesota State Board of Health. A shocking seventeen of the twenty cases had resulted from Terro Ant Killer. Of these, five had been children. The survey prompted me to publish articles on the sources, symptoms, and signs of arsenic intoxication in 1982 and 1983 in two well-known and widely read medical journals.

In 1988 an employee of the Environmental Protection Agency contacted me and asked if I would be a witness at a judicial hearing to determine if the registrations for arsenic-containing ant killers should be canceled. At the hearing in Washington, DC, I presented additional cases of poisoning by Terro Ant Killer collected by the Poison Control Center at the Texas Tech Health Sciences Center. Based on testimony from a number of medical experts, the court observed the problem with sodium arsenate ant killers was not localized to a given region of the country but was widespread. It also confirmed that less toxic substances than arsenic existed for killing ants.

After a thorough investigation by the EPA, a long and impressive judicial hearing, the Administrative Law Court acted. On May 22, 1989, the registrations for arsenic-containing ant killers in the United States were canceled. While the ant killers today may bear the same names, they now contain less risky active ingredients such as boric acid.

*Chapter 6*

# THE THEODORA CONSULT

*Just as dogs love to chew bones, the mind loves to get its teeth into problems.*

That's why it does crossword puzzles and builds atom bombs.
—Eckhart Tolle

During my professional career, I performed tens of thousands of neurological evaluations. In medical shorthand, I refer to these as consults, for example, as brain tumor consults, multiple sclerosis consults, and memory disorder consults. When speaking to friends and colleagues about the consultation described in this chapter, I found the encounter required no such modifier. It became known merely as "The Theodora Consult." No other neurological conundrum challenged me quite in the same fashion.

"When did your walking go haywire?" I asked the young man who had recently been admitted to Ward 2C of the Minneapolis VA Hospital. I sat at his bedside in my below-the-knee white faculty coat with black bag resting on his bedside table.

The neurology wards totaled eighty-two beds equally divided between Ward 2C and Ward 2D. Each ward typically had large rooms of six to ten beds, although a few private ones existed. The multibed rooms had drapes separating the beds, which allowed for at least an illusion of privacy. Between drawn curtains my team of trainees huddled, their waist-length or knee-length white coats signaling their various levels of training.

The patient cosseted at the center of our attention was Billy Stephens, a twenty-eight-year-old man, admitted the previous evening for walking difficulty. He wore VA-issue pajamas, sandals, and a thin brown-striped dressing gown. Large windows flooded the room with a soft, natural light.

"I told Doctor Swenson last night," he said, gesturing with his grimy fingernail toward the intern. "I wanted to go see *Star Wars*. As the stars flashed, the music came up, and the words rolled on the screen—'In a galaxy far, far away'—I felt real strange. I was walking down the aisle. My legs got wobbly, and I fell into a seat."

"What happened next?" I asked.

"Well, watched the movie. It was good, too. When the movie was over, I got up to leave. I learned then I couldn't walk right. I staggered up the aisle. My buddies freaked, and since I was a veteran and all, they hauled me to the emergency room here."

It was 1977, during the hot and humid dog days of a Minnesota summer. The mosquitoes had by then grown to extraordinary size and appetite, providing veracity to the aphorism that the Minnesota state bird was actually the mosquito. I was an instructor at the University of Minnesota and served as a staff neurologist at the Veteran's Administration Hospital. My clinical assignment that month was a ward service, consisting of around twenty-five patients, a neurological resident, two interns, and four medical students.

"Did you have numbness, pain, or weakness?" I asked the slightly built veteran lying in the hospital bed.

"Everything was normal, just couldn't stay on top of my legs." Billy had a chopped look to his short black hair, unruly eyebrows, and a thin, wiry frame. He had completed high school, enlisted in the army, and served a hitch in Vietnam.

Following his discharge, Billy had joined a traveling Christian ministry based somewhere within the Bible Belt. During the warmer seasons, he moved from city to city, putting up and taking down the ministry's tent, furnishing the podium and the pulpit, directing religious or curiosity seekers to their chairs, and never failing on cue to pass the collection plates.

Earlier I had learned Billy's medical history from the intern and heard briefer comments from the resident. Billy Stephens's unique symptom onset and unusual walking had perplexed both intern and resident.

"Well, let's get to it, Mr. Stephens. Show me how you walk." A concerned look came over Stephens's face. He gingerly sat up in bed and slowly hung his legs off the side. He then slipped carefully off the side of the bed but maintained a firm, white-knuckled grasp on the bed rail. Billy stood quietly for a few seconds. While his feet remained in place on the floor, his torso then began to weave to and fro with increasing excursions. This continued for a few seconds before he reluctantly turned loose of the bed rail. With limited assistance from Doctor Swenson, he began to walk across the ward. Billy lurched from side to side, and at one point a medical student rushed to prevent him from falling. But Billy proved adept at catching himself and did not fall, instead grabbing for support at a nearby pillar. This process repeated itself with Billy righting himself on a bed, chair, and wall. Each time, he would slowly straighten up, gather his fortitude, grudgingly let go of his support, and veer off wildly in another direction.

"See, Doctor, not getting any better," Billy interjected at several points. He displayed a perplexed expression on his face. I thanked him for his bravery and asked that he be helped back into his bed.

My entourage, several with stethoscopes bobbing casually around their necks, departed the ward. We trooped toward a nearby conference room close to the elevators. I noticed while walking down the hallway the distinctive and faintly unpleasant astringent scent that always permeated the hospital.

*The cleaning products must have come from the lowest bidder.*

I led the group into a conference room not far from the ward. All took their seats in front of an old green chalkboard whose tray overflowed with white chalk powder. I asked in what I hoped was a professorial voice, "Has anyone seen a gait like Mr. Stephens's?" I looked around the group and viewed shaking heads and blank faces.

Finally Rory Magee, a medical student, spoke up. "Last week I saw a man with ataxia due to alcoholism." Rory was trying to be helpful and obviously proud to use his recently learned medical term for uncoordinated movement.

"Did the man with the alcoholic injury to his cerebellum walk like Mr. Stephens?" I addressed this question to the group but focused in particular on Rory, the curly-haired medical student.

"No, he didn't. He walked with his feet wide apart and helped balance by putting his arms out. Mr. Stephens had his feet close together. He lurched from side to side but surprised me by catching himself and never falling. If the alcoholic man had staggered that way, he'd have ended up on the floor in a one-man dog pile."

*This student has the potential to be a neurologist!*

"An excellent observation, Rory. Has anyone else seen patients with walking problems due to peripheral nerve injury, spinal cord disease, brain-stem injury, cerebellar injury, or cerebral disease who walked like Mr. Stephens?" I looked about the room at my baffled ward team. Most were shaking their heads. I observed several vacant expressions.

"Well, what does that tell us?" I asked, waiting a few seconds for the question to penetrate before answering my own question. "Tells us, his walking problems are inconsistent with injury to the nervous system." The room fell completely silent with all eyes on me.

*Say, this teaching is fun.*

"His walking problem is not neurological. It's likely psychogenic," I said, hoping to sound wise and dramatic.

"You mean he's faking it?" asked Christy Brown, a lively female medical student whose career goal was to become a pediatrician.

"No, not necessarily, Christy. If he were feigning, we would call it malingering. If his symptoms stem from his subconscious, we refer to it as hysteria. Admittedly, teasing out malingering from hysteria can be tricky. But based on a lack of clear financial gain, I doubt Mr. Stephens is malingering." I saw heads nod, so I decided to expand further on the concept.

"Unusual symptoms of hysteria result from the subconscious. The patient is unaware emotional aspects drive the disordered walking, movement, or sensory abnormality. We will in all likelihood end up calling this hysteria in Mr. Stephens's situation, and refer to it specifically as a hysteric gait."

"Is this the same as a conversion reaction?" asked Christy, who had completed her psychiatry rotation.

"The psychiatrists use a different classification system and refer to such mind-based symptoms as conversion reactions," I said. "No matter what we call it, hysterical reaction or conversion disorder, the symptoms spring from deep within the unconscious mind and suggest unresolved psychological needs."

"Who gets hysteria?" asked another medical student.

"Usually hysteric symptoms occur in people who see the world in black-and-white terms, are usually poorly educated, and deal poorly with their emotions."

"Guess that's why the CT scan was normal," said Doctor Swenson, an intern with blue eyes and long blond hair. He paused and then asked, "Can we just tell him his problems are all in his head?"

"Afraid it's more complicated than that," I replied. "We must first learn what psychological advantage he obtains from his symptoms, and then figure out a way to work him through it. We will find a way to make his walking problem inconvenient by removing his psychological gain. We will devise a face-saving way for Billy to rid himself of his walking problem."

The discussion that followed centered on gaining more information about Billy Stephens's life. For the next several days, we would determine what psychological factors existed that could either confirm or refute our clinical suspicion of hysteria. I instructed the ward team that Mr. Stephens's problem was as real for him as a stroke or brain tumor. As his physicians, we needed to maintain his confidence and continue interviewing him for relevant information.

After rounds that day, I felt satisfaction for recognizing Stephens's walking problem for what it was. I understood my diagnosis had resulted from having seen other patients with hysterical gaits, as well as having dealt with other neurological symptoms of hysteria.

Billy's case gave me a greater appreciation for my mentors for having taught the peculiarities of different types of abnormal walking. I felt particularly indebted to the chairman of neurology and residency director, Doctor A. B. Baker. While widely recognized as a world expert in stroke and for having established the American Academy of Neurology, he also possessed amazing insights into psychogenic illnesses. As such, the University of Minnesota had become a referral site for patients from all over the country suffering such illnesses, allowing his trainees to gain valuable experience with these disorders.

A. B. Baker, the showman that he was, had developed intricate procedures for working patients through their hysteric symptoms. When the secondary gain had been identified and removed and when Doctor Baker had determined the patients were psychologically receptive to letting go of their symptoms, only then would he move into the treatment phase.

With much fanfare and with the assistance of his capable and theatrical Nurse Clipper, Doctor Baker would arrive ceremoniously with his "black box." This highly touted device generated a limited amount of harmless electrical current. The treatment consisted of manipulation of the controls and varying placement of the electrodes. To great advantage Doctor Baker, the professor, projected authority and confidence. Many patients after receiving the black box treatment experienced miraculous cures and rose up from their sick beds to leave the hospital.

These demonstrations proved dramatic and at times comedic, requiring all in attendance to maintain sober facial expressions.

Over the next several days (everything in those days moved slower in medicine, particularly at VA hospitals), we learned more about Billy Stephens's psychological makeup.

One morning on rounds, Doctor Swenson offered, "I learned from Billy's friend that Billy was bored with his job. He wanted more challenging work, worthy of greater respect." The friend said Billy had been vying for the attention of the evangelist but had proved too insignificant in the organization to gain her attention.

Christy added, "I learned that Billy barely graduated from high school. You might say he escaped through the back door with his diploma. He joined the army but never moved beyond the rank of private. Served in Vietnam. Did not see conflict, based in large camps, mostly fixing equipment. Billy didn't get into any serious trouble, but was never material for higher rank."

A psychological evaluation stated Billy had little insight into his feelings or the feelings of others. He was described as "psychologically unsophisticated." The report detailed several emotionally charged episodes from Billy's past in which he had reacted poorly.

Our understanding of Billy's psychological makeup increased. It was clear he had unresolved emotional issues, thought about life in black-and-white terms, had limited education, had symptoms that began in an emotionally charged environment, and had unmet needs for higher status. Nevertheless, Billy had no insight into the nature of his symptoms and no perceptible financial gain; examination tricks designed to trip up malingering had failed to do so. All of our findings pointed to Billy having a hysterical illness. In recognition of all this, I formulated our treatment plan. The following morning's rounds would be our first opportunity to put the initial portion of the plan into action.

The next morning when all the team was clustered around

Billy, I began. "Mr. Stephens, your doctors have spent a great amount of time pondering your walking problem," I said solemnly. Stephens leaned in, listening carefully to this, the final formulation of his illness. He furrowed his brow and his unruly eyebrows peaked.

"Well, doctor, what's wrong with me?" he asked tentatively, his dark eyes studying me carefully.

"Mr. Stephens, I regret we have not found any specifically treatable illness. Your problem is beyond the realm of our understanding in medicine. We know that you cannot work because of your walking problems, nor even function normally in society." I said all this with a sympathetic tone.

"Well, what's going to happen to me?" Billy asked pleadingly, as he shifted restlessly in his bed. I paused briefly to avoid competing with the hospital's overhead speaker system that just then was announcing a special cut-rate sale in the canteen on cartons of unfiltered cigarettes.

"I am afraid we must place you in a VA domiciliary hospital. There the nurses will help you with your needs, and you will have companionship with other disabled veterans." To make the situation more awful in Billy's eyes, I provided a short list of several domiciliary hospitals, each located in forsaken, out-of-the-way places.

A look of dismay came over Billy Stephens's face. His shoulders slumped. He appeared to implode before our eyes. Whatever deep psychological reasons caused his hysteric gait, my approach was not what his psyche craved.

"How long will I be in that place?" Billy asked. His voice was tinged with hopefulness.

"Well, likely for the rest of your life." With this comment, Billy deflated further like a punctured inner tube. Christy edged closer to the bed and placed a comforting arm around Billy.

*Nice touch, Christy.*

"Jeeesus," Billy exclaimed. "Nothing you can do at all? A domiciliary? That's where old vets go to die."

I paused several counts before responding in what I hoped

was a sage-sounding voice. "Mr. Stephens, I have one more idea, but it is, well, it is still highly, uh, uh, *experimental*."

"Tell me," Billy said with urgency in his voice. Billy moved in closer and regained his look of rapt attention.

"There is a new, investigational electrical treatment that just might work—that is, if you are willing to try it."

"Absolutely!" he shouted out in a too-loud voice. "By all means, Doctor. When can we begin?"

"Well, it will take time to arrange the treatment room, equipment, and nurse. Let's wait until tomorrow morning to start your treatment," I said. "In the meantime, you take it easy. You know, Billy," I added, while patting the back of his hand, "the more I think about it, the more I think this treatment will be highly effective and should fix you up." With this statement I had given the positive suggestion that his cure was imminent.

After rounds that day, I scheduled the treatment room on Ward 2C for the following morning. I then scurried over to the university to borrow Doctor Baker's black box. On my return I spoke at length to the ward's charge nurse, Molly Anderson, a bouncy brunette with flashing brown eyes. She seemed excited to play her role in our psychological intervention. In the privacy of my office, Molly and I choreographed our treatment of Billy. I thought Molly's personality would serve well in our mock scientific treatment.

After having planted my positive suggestion, I felt the passage of a little time was needed for the idea of a cure to permeate Billy's psyche. Billy's confused psychology needed time to reequilibrate and for him subconsciously to recognize his disordered gait no longer provided him with any advantage. My confidence was growing that Billy would respond favorably to a face-saving method for ridding him of his psychogenic ataxia. I looked forward to banishing his walking problem and anticipated in addition a dramatic clinical demonstration for my trainees.

The ward team had kept Billy's confidence, a necessary ingredient to make the plan effective. As a group, they would further promote the black box's remarkable healing properties. All that was left for me in the morning was to artfully place the electrodes, spin the dials, utter a few unintelligible Latin phrases, have Molly strut her stuff, and await Billy's dramatic transformation from ataxic state to normal mobility.

I felt my excitement growing. I was jazzed by the exciting prospect that lay ahead. But it was at that point that my well-laid plans hurtled wildly and unpredictably off course. And like a bolt of lightning from the sky, I never saw it coming.

Billy's traveling ministry had experienced a profitable run in the Twin Cities and had camped there longer than initially anticipated. During his hospitalization, Billy had maintained contact with his friend, a fellow handyman at the ministry. By pure coincidence his buddy had persuaded the traveling evangelist to visit a lonely Billy that very afternoon.

I was working at my desk when I saw a heavy-set, red-robed woman adorned by copious gold jewelry, large gold hoop earrings, and bouffant, peroxide-blond hair stroll by my office door. To be sure, the middle-aged woman's appearance was not the usual visitor to our wards, and I assumed she must be the evangelist. Slightly behind her walked a wispy-looking young man. They headed in the direction of Ward 2C.

I stepped from my office and said, "Good afternoon. May I help you find someone?"

"Why, yes, I am Sister Theodora," she said in a majestic tone after slowly turning and gazing disdainfully upon me. "I seek Billy Stephens. He serves me at the Worldwide Christian Apostolic Ministries, or as we call it, World-CAM. And I need him back at work, right away." She said this dismissively and evinced an uncompromising demeanor, as if she were accustomed to having people respond promptly to her directives.

"I am Doctor Hutton, the attending neurologist for Mr. Stephens. I would be glad to direct you to him." I saw Sister Theodora's face brighten at the unexpected opportunity to gain information, especially, I thought, about how fast I could get him back to work at World-CAM. Sister Theodora stepped in closer, and I noticed she stood no more than five feet tall and was nearly as wide as she was tall.

"Well, how's Billy doing?" Sister Theodora asked. She wore heavy black mascara and red rouge, and a heavy gold cross was hanging around her thick neck. She smelled faintly of incense.

"I am afraid his walking problem is no better," I said. "But we will begin his treatment in the morning. We are getting everything set up now. Hopefully he will be back at work very soon."

"Is that the fastest you can move? I am in great need of Billy's services to assist me in doing the Lord's work, *tonight*," she said grandly.

I carefully observed Sister Theodora. While having a charismatic personality, her interaction with me smacked of haughtiness. She took in my limited information and appeared to consider it only momentarily. Little else of substance transpired between us before I directed her to Billy's room.

I continued to watch after her as she trundled down the shiny green linoleum hallway with her sycophant trailing behind. I could not resist walking after her as far as the nurses' station, from where I could feign review of a chart but, in reality, monitor her interactions with Billy. I saw her approach Billy's bedside and the two exchanged pleasantries. The squat, red-clad Sister Theodora stood regally at Billy's bedside.

I had just turned to leave a few minutes later when Sister Theodora began in a remarkably loud voice to recite an incantation. I heard a hush fall over the usual din on the ward and turned to observe patients and staff craning their heads in her direction. I noticed Sister Theodora smile faintly before placing her chubby hands on the sides of Billy's head. She pushed at his temples like his head was a giant tube of toothpaste. I saw Billy startle at first, then sit up, as if at attention. Sister Theodora then dropped her hands and began to stride purposefully around Billy's bed, finding difficulty fitting between the head of the bed and the wall. She then summoned in a loud voice the celestial healing powers to bear on Billy. All the while she continued her unusual, dissonant chant.

Sister Theodora at last stopped circling and stood resplendently in front of Billy. She gazed upon him with a wild look on her face, raised her arms in supplication, and sternly ordered, "Billy, get out of your bed and with the help of God Almighty, *walk!*"

He straightened up further in bed and immediately scooted to the side of the bed. Billy hopped off his mattress and without hesitation walked unerringly across the ward. I saw his young face radiate pleasure and relief. His self-confidence at that moment struck me as sufficient to walk a tightrope across Niagara Falls. Sister Theodora's countenance never failed to project anything but utter certainty.

As I watched all this, I felt a mix of emotions. On the one hand, I felt like a dog whose bone had just been stolen by the neighbor's thieving hound. On the other hand, I recognized my careful staging had facilitated this remarkable and unfolding drama.

*Does it make any difference where the credit goes for Billy's improvement?*

Soon thereafter I departed for home. When I arrived there, I found myself largely inattentive to Trudy and Andy. My mind was still thinking about Billy and the squatty evangelist. I slept fitfully that night but awoke the next morning with a clearer mind.

When I returned to work, I learned that Billy Stephens had demanded and received his discharge from the hospital the night before. He had gathered his possessions, waved good-bye to the staff, and departed for the ministry's encampment.

"Looks like Sister Theodora beat us to the punch," I responded lightheartedly on rounds that morning. I said this while our medical team sat grumpily in the conference room, studying Doctor Baker's black box for which we now had no need.

"What do you think will happen to Billy Stephens?" asked the towheaded Doctor Swenson.

"No way to know for sure," I said. "But I suspect Billy may have predictable relapses, if you know what I mean."

"You mean Billy might become a regular at the revival?" asked Christy.

"Christy, I would not be surprised if he becomes a cornerstone of the good Sister's show. At the very least, I am sure Sister Theodora will point out in her booming voice at every opportunity how she cured a man when medical science and the doctors had failed. But we have to remember that our scientific perspective is not the only one. Sister Theodora will maintain that Billy's dramatic healing was a miracle from her beseeching of the Almighty."

Now decades later when reflecting on a career in which I treated dozens of patients with hysterical illnesses, I find myself considering "miracles" differently. I wonder how many purported miracles are phenomena poorly understood by overly simplistic observers. How many of the cures at revivals are in fact psychogenic illnesses that give way to the power of authoritative suggestion?

I suspect claims of so-called miracles have decreased over the centuries in the face of improved scientific understanding and greater reasoning abilities. In recent centuries, medical science may have even altered the very meaning of miracles. Heart transplants, joint replacements, and artificial kidneys are often referred to as "medical miracles." But is it not easier for many to attribute unexplained and confusing happenings to miracles rather than to poor understanding of scientific processes?

I have come to believe that miracles reside in the eye of the beholder. One person's miracle may be another's scientific advance or broader understanding. The conflict between science and religion bothers me less than it used to. I arrived at the realization that the primary importance was to ensure people get better, regardless of method.

"Doctor Hutton, are you irritated by having spent so much time understanding Mr. Stephens's illness and making his symptoms uncomfortable, only to have the evangelist scoop you?" Christy asked. While her eyes showed mirth, she also asked the question with an engaging sincerity.

I paused and smiled before answering. "Who knows, Christy, maybe if Sister Theodora remains in the Twin Cities, I will consult her again. The best treatment, after all, for a hysterical illness is a hysterical treatment. In terms of effectiveness, I have to agree that Sister Theodora's approach was no better or worse than our own. Sister Theodora and those of us in medicine just view the world in different ways."

## Chapter 7

# ROLLING THE DICE: CROSS-COUNTRY MOTORING WITH THE WORLD'S MOST INCORRIGIBLE DALMATIAN

*Humor is the greatest thing, the saving thing. The minute it crops up, all our irritation and resentments slip away, and a sunny spirit takes their place.*

—Mark Twain

Let me begin my tale at the outset of my twelve-hundred-mile cross-country journey. If this road trip were compared to a particular space trip, then it would best parallel the ill-fated Apollo 13 mission. My trajectory began arcing toward disaster when I glanced in the rearview mirror to bid a farewell to Minneapolis only instead to find the reflection of a dog's maw, drooling like Niagara Falls. *Houston, we have a problem!*

In November of 1981, our dog Dice and I departed Minneapolis for Lubbock, Texas. Trudy, Andy, and our toddler, Katie, stayed behind in Bloomington. While cowardice comes to mind, my wife claims to this day their departure had to await the up-coming school break—a highly suspect notion in my opinion.

At eighty pounds, Dice fit the backseat of our compact car like Shaquille O'Neal would fit the cockpit of an F-16. With each bounce of the car, his nearly all white head would impact the roof. This caused me no great alarm as Dice's brain seemed the least vulnerable portion of his anatomy.

Dice and I barreled southward on I-35 past dormant fields tucked in for the winter. The whirring sound of snow tires on pavement blended with Dice's metronome-like panting, lulling me into an unfortunate sense of security. The hound and I had departed Minneapolis ahead of a blizzard that would soon cover the state with several feet of ice and snow. Minnesota lore had it that the weather consisted of nine months of frigid winter, followed by three months of hard sledding! After ten years on the tundra with its ten thousand mostly frozen lakes, I remain convinced this portrayal was far too charitable.

Our car hummed southward through Faribault, Minnesota, and continued south. Dice, who by then was loudly snoring, would intermittently jolt the back of my seat with his restless hind legs.

Before reaching Iowa, my canine companion stirred, rose groggily to his feet, and extended his mopey countenance over my shoulder. Dice had crossed eyes, a feature that made me uncomfortable, never being quite sure if he was looking at me or not.

Years before when selecting the puppy, the breeder had assured us that Dice would grow to no larger than forty-five pounds—false advertising at its best. At maturity Dice's Brobdingnagian-like body bore scant resemblance to the breeder's prediction or to the cuddly puppies my son had fallen in love with in *101 Dalmatians*. Dice had few spots, a scoring demerit by the American Kennel Club. However, this imperfection blanched in comparison to his indisputable, unassailable lack of canine IQ.

To be numbingly honest, Dice was light-years away from being a smart dog. The heavily inbred Dalmatian bears a well-deserved reputation as being "a slow learner." While Dalmatians may look regal atop fire engines and Anheuser-Busch beer wagons, the Dalmatian in terms of smarts ranks as the Elmer Fudd of the dog world. The befuddled thinking of this breed makes cocker spaniels and Chihuahuas appear as candidates for PhDs. Come to think of it, iguanas with special needs may be smarter than was our Dice.

While rarely task-focused, Dice possessed stupendous energy. Watching Dice galloping figure eights in the snow and effortlessly jumping hedges had been for me a neck-tingling spectator sport. But Dice's exuberance, coupled with his non-existent self-control, made the extended road trip to Lubbock worrisome in the extreme.

Anticipating this and being a resourceful physician (read: desperate), I penned a prescription for Valium in the name of (ahem) Mr. D. Hutton of Bloomington, Minnesota. Each morning of the road trip, one tablet would be pushed down the old doggie gullet. In addition to the calming effect, the medicine had a side effect unmentioned in my *Physician's Desk Reference*. Dice began to drool like the Trevi Fountain.

Admittedly, Dice had a few admirable traits. He protected his family, even if at times mistaken about who represented the good guys and who the bad guys. He also possessed a fearsome growl that promised security for the family when I was working late. But to be sure, Dice's main benefit was his ability to make us laugh. We often had erupted in gut-grabbing guffaws over Dice's wiggly, wayward antics and his unbridled enthusiasm for life.

In the overfilled backseat, my cross-eyed Dice sat bent over with his long, pink tongue hanging out like an emergency slide from a Boeing 767. He appeared mellow, no doubt in part from the Valium. Also, traveling in a car was his favorite activity, followed closely by his retrieval of and attempts to bury postmen in our front yard.

My soggy shoulder, courtesy of Dice, helped distract me from other creeping anxieties. I was feeling deeply ambivalent about our move. After all, I was leaving behind friendships bonded by childbirths and the shared penury of the young married set. These warm relationships would prove difficult, if not impossible, to replace. I would miss these wonderful, winterized sons and daughters of Scandinavians and Germans with whom we had enjoyed affirmation and abundant laughter.

As I drove onward, I began to hear a rasping noise mixed in with the whirring sound of the snow tires. I could not identify the sound. Soon a Mac Davis song, "Texas in My Rearview Mirror," crowded out the whirring and rasping noises. Our friends, thoroughly mystified by our decision to depart Minnesota, had given us the Mac Davis tape at our going-away party. In the central song, Davis croons, "Happiness was Lubbock, Texas, in my rearview mirror." We suspected they had not so subtly cast doubt upon our decision to move to Lubbock, as they had played the song around fifty times. I recalled their incredulous looks in response to our explanations. Why, they asked, would anyone wish to depart the land of ten thousand (*mostly frozen*) lakes for arid West Texas? *You think, just maybe, they believe we're making a mistake?*

But ahead lay not only a parched landscape and slow-talking strangers, but also the promise of an associate professor's position at a developing medical school. Opportunity beckoned! *Move west, young man, move west!*

The challenge of my new job, accepted in a fit of homesickness for our native Texas, was merely to conjure up a neurological clinical, teaching, and research program where none had ever existed at a struggling medical school established not to train specialists but to churn out primary care physicians. Piece of cake, right?

Prior to my departure from Minneapolis, Trudy, with a look of concern, imparted some final directions. She began her presentation with, "Since you *only* have to begin a job and care for *only* one dog."

Given this lax schedule of mine, Trudy had determined that I should examine the primary and secondary schools in Lubbock. Then I should settle on which ones had the most rigorous academic standards, boasted the best teaching staffs, and provided the greatest assurance that their schools warranted our precocious and gifted offspring. In addition, the schools must be located near good shopping. Following this, I should snag a close by, cute, well-landscaped home in a good neighborhood for not very much money. *Why not ask for a Hollywood hair stylist and a free membership at the country club?* Her challenge was clearly an invitation for failure with an unstated penalty of my obtaining a long-term sleeping berth on the couch.

While ruminating on friends left behind, a challenging new job, and the quest for housing to meet Trudy's high standards, I cruised through rolling Iowa farmlands, turned west across the hilly terrain of northern Missouri, and eventually passed over the state line into aptly named Prairie Village, Kansas. There Dice and I would overnight with my aunt Grace, whom my siblings and I called Nonnie.

My seventy-five-year-old, gray-haired, sub-five-foot aunt was so slight as to be at risk in a Kansas windstorm. The widow Nonnie lived on a quiet residential street in a subdued green cottage with black shutters. I bounced the car over the low curb into Nonnie's narrow driveway. The deepening shadows of late evening had set in. In my enthusiasm to greet Nonnie, I failed to leash up the Dalmatian. Dice slipped out of the car and unloaded ten gallons on a nearby tree, no doubt stunting its growth for years. Dice then pivoted from the tree and like a Stinger missile headed for my Munchkin-like aunt. While loving animals in the abstract, Nonnie suffered a long-standing phobia of any dog larger than a Pomeranian.

"Crikey," I heard Nonnie shriek in her high-pitched voice, while she furiously crawfished back onto the front porch. Her repeated cries of alarm rebounded up and down the block of peaceful-looking, cookie-cutter homes.

"Stop, Dice, oh, PLEEEEEEEASE stop!" I screamed. The dog briefly halted his charge, closed his eyes, and extended his muscular neck. He began a series of bellows—long, mournful howls. Up and down the street, porch lights began to switch on. Just before I could reach him, he again dashed toward my, by then, cowering aunt.

On seeing Dice's flat-out charge, my aunt's facial expression transformed from welcoming to Frisbee-eyed. Dice leapt onto the small porch and drove Nonnie back into the corner. There he stood on his hind legs, bracketing her against the shingled wall. He looked like Marmaduke, towering over my diminutive aunt. I was only slightly relieved when he chose not to drag her from the porch and plant her in the nearest flowerbed.

Then a further surprise happened. Nonnie, with unexpected dexterity, no doubt fueled by cresting fear, ducked under his extended front leg. Foolishly believing she could escape the crazed hound, she opened the front door and slipped into the house. A look of dumbfounded recognition came over Dice, as novel territory beckoned like a giant beefsteak from inside. Momentarily he shivered with anticipation and then exploded through the still-closing door.

Nonnie's home was tastefully decorated with quaint antique furniture, rare china, and porcelain treasures. As Dice bolted in, my hands rose reflexively to my head. I gave an anguished cry, beseeching my out-of-control dog to halt.

"No, Dice. Please, Dice, come back. Oh God, don't!" By then several of the neighbors were out their lighted front doors with hands on hips, scowling in our direction.

My urgent plea to Dice was ignored. I doubted it had even registered within his crazed brain. Fearsome sounds soon began to emanate from the house. I heard glass crashing and furniture overturning. Dice's muffled wailing wafted from the house. My aunt gave several high-pitched exclamations. I knew if left undeterred, Dice would soon convert a peaceful, well-ordered home into a doggie demolition derby.

I threw open the door and raced full bore into the house. I viewed the spotted one careening from room to room. Dice's crossed eyes and flapping tongue gave him a demonic look. I chased him through the living room, just missed him in the kitchen when he outmaneuvered me, and finally cornered him in the dining room next to the china cabinet. After a diving tackle and a spirited tussle under the cherry French-Provincial table amongst a forest of Queen Anne chair legs, I drug a struggling Dice across the highly polished hardwood floor, through the back door, and onto an enclosed back porch. There with my chest heaving, I determined he could safely spend the night. My only concern then was whether my aunt would be willing to relinquish the butcher's knife she clasped in her hand.

That night both my sleep and my conscience were troubled. By the next morning Nonnie had seemingly calmed herself and was speaking to me. For this I was pleased. *This proves either the strength of blood ties or the curative powers of strong sherry.*

After breakfast served on surviving Wedgwood china plates, I mumbled my umpteenth apology and offered loving goodbyes. After a visit like that, there was not much else I could say. I declined a small sack of doggie treats, suspicious that Nonnie had laced them with strychnine, then loaded the already tranquilized Dice into the car. I could not have exited Prairie Village any faster had Bonnie and Clyde been chasing me with submachine guns. I knew further overnight stays with family or friends were far too risky and that despite the expense, Dice and I in the future would stay at motels.

The car hummed along Highway 71 and was Texas-bound. In the passenger side of the front seat rode my black bag with my name embossed in gold. I felt a deep sense of pride over this gift received at the conclusion of my medical school training. Within it were various instruments I would need to examine patients at my new position at the Texas Tech School of Medicine. I did not know how fond I would become of these independent-minded West Texans.

The worrisome grating sound again drifted from the back part of the car. I assumed the noise came from the heavily treaded snow tires being driven over dry pavement.

Hours later I stopped for lunch at a McDonald's drive-through. After I paid the tab, the attendant tried to pass the food sack through the car window. Dice lunged, his gleaming canines falling inches short of the attendant's hand. I reached out and grabbed the food sack, stomped on the accelerator, peeled out, and prayed the hamburger flipper would be too distracted to record my license plate. *I wonder if dog mauling falls under worker's comp.*

I later stopped at a tranquil town park and secured Dice via a leash to the bumper. I placed his dog bowls before him. Dice then proceeded to wolf down a can of dog food, a large portion of kibble, and leftovers from a large burger, fries, and vanilla shake before lapping up three quarters of a bowl of water. His ravenous appetite was no longer a surprise for me. Although Dice's voraciousness was notorious, his digestive tract seemed destined for epic status. *Maybe Dice could be an advertising pitch-dog for supersizing.*

While still a pup, Dice once had stolen two pecan pies off the kitchen counter and consumed both inside of a minute. Making matters worse, my in-laws had just completed the thousand-mile car trip from Dallas to Minneapolis with the pies uncomfortably underfoot. Within minutes of carrying the famous family recipe pies into the house and nanoseconds after human eyes were diverted, our Thanksgiving dessert resided within our dog's cavernous stomach. Surprise, disbelief, and anger had sprung from my usually genteel in-laws. In subsequent years my mother-in-law could never again look at Dice without scowling and complaining about "that pie-poaching puppy." Dice just seemed to have his own way of bringing out grudges in people.

Another time, Dice stole a roasted chicken off the dining room table and ate it, bones and all, without so much as belching. And at the completion of my residency, Trudy served up two heavenly steaks for our celebratory dinner. Steak had proven to be a commodity as rare on a house officer's salary as fricasseed wildebeest. While I tucked into my meal and Trudy briefly returned to the kitchen to retrieve the vegetables, Dice unobtrusively filched her beef.

"Have you seen my rib eye?" Trudy asked on her return.

"Nope, you bring it in yet?" I said still looking down at my plate. After several seconds of contemplation, our eyes were in unison drawn toward Dice like metal filings to a magnet. We made eye contact, after which he skulked from the dining area, licking his larcenous lips.

A simple rib eye was no match for Dice. He had, after all, been known to consume shoes, buckles and all. But once, his ravenous ways almost did him in. When wolfing down pieces of leftover meat, he ate with such haste that he inhaled a chunk of meat. To my horror, he began to wheeze and gasp for air. I chased after him and found him collapsed within our front entry hall.

My medical instincts took over. While straddling Dice, I performed the Heimlich maneuver. The meat popped up like a cork from a champagne bottle and flew halfway across the room. Dice sucked in a mighty gulp of air and proceeded to pounce on the meat, chew it briefly, swallow, and as if nothing had happened, return to his food bowl to vacuum up the remaining scraps. Now traveling in the car with the *Canis familiaris* slobbering onto my shoulder and panting his stinky breath, I for the one-thousandth time questioned the wisdom of ever having performed the rescue maneuver.

The miles rolled by. Eventually Dice began to whine. Suspecting he needed a break, I stopped at a roadside park in eastern Oklahoma. I leashed up Dice and looked forward to stretching my legs.

Parenthetically, it should be noted here that Dice had not succeeded at Sven and Lena's Dog Obedience School located in Bloomington, Minnesota. He had not merely been a poor student but the sole dog in three decades to be booted from the obedience school. His failure followed what I considered, at least by Dice's standards, a fairly minor infraction. He had, during the course of the evening, humped a pink miniature poodle, terrorized a beagle, pilfered a dozen White Castle burgers, and hoisted his leg on Lena's beaded designer jeans. Such incidents were commonplace for our irredeemable Dice. Lena and Sven thought differently.

Sven really got worked up over it. He had yelled in his singsong English, "You get dat damned dawg from my school, and never, ever should return it." I was surprised at Sven. I had not seen that much emotion in a Minnesotan since Fran Tarkenton retired from the Vikings. I rationalized that Sven probably was upset over the loss of his bland, stamp-sized, tasteless burgers, and I offered to buy him a brand-new sack full to appease him. *Those Scandinavian types never had developed a taste for properly spiced foods.* Getting the boot from Sven and Lena's was not such a big deal, since Dice had not learned even basic skills, such as walking on a leash.

To return to my troubled cross-country sojourn, Dice, on jumping out of the car, spied a tawny cat lurking among the bushes. He immediately sprinted off, hitting the end of his leash like a tarpon striking a lure and causing me whiplash. Despite coughing from constriction of his windpipe, Dice proceeded to grind inexorably onward like a miniature Sherman tank with spots. His muscles rippled and his feet dug paw divots. His eyes bugged out, but his muzzle bore a look of fierce determination.

I planted my heels in the moist grass but had difficulty gaining purchase. I desperately clutched at the leash, knowing that if Dice escaped, I would have unfathomable difficulty retrieving him. How could I tell Andy and Katie that I had lost their pet?

As I leaned against the leash like a water skier on a towrope, I became vaguely aware of cars slowing and a few exiting the highway. Several eighteen-wheelers had also left the highway and amid a whooshing of air brakes parked alongside this unfolding man-versus-dog drama. After a few more minutes of futile struggling, I glanced up to see grizzled truckers and fresh-faced families gaping at us through their windshields.

One trucker was laughing so hard he spit out his cigar and his baseball cap toppled from his head.

The gawkers witnessed a spot-challenged Dalmatian pulling a hapless man who was foot-plowing furrows through the roadside park. Dice, in his wild pursuit of the cat, had pulled me across thorny bushes and nearly the length of the parking lot. Not until the spotted demon pulled me over a cement bench was I able to break his momentum. His progress halted, he forsook the cat pursuit. Needless to say, the Oklahoma park-plowing incident was not my proudest moment.

Using a cookie, I bribed Dice to load back into the car. We pulled out of the park, leaving my embarrassment behind, and soon merged onto the Will Rogers Freeway. By then my patience with Dice was as thin as one-ply toilet tissue. The shadows were lengthening just as my eyelids began to droop. I drove into Tulsa and stopped at a diner.

An hour later I departed the restaurant sated but even drowsier than before. I was intent on finding a pillow—and soon. Discouraging motel signs trumpeted no dogs allowed. I turned onto Interstate 40, heading westward toward Oklahoma City.

I found no overnight accommodations between Tulsa and Oklahoma City. On arriving in the capital city of Oklahoma, I crept along the motel strip, searching for an available room. I stopped and inquired at several. Motel after motel prohibited dogs. *My God, what do these Oklahomans have against dogs!* Finally, I stopped at a motel on the western outskirts, believing it to be my last hope prior to having to drive to Amarillo.

Seeing no notice proscribing dogs, I entered the motel office. "Got a room?"

"You're lucky, just one left," said the man from the subcontinent in heavily accented English. He handed me a key across a scratched glass counter. A strong curry odor drifted from the back room.

I completed the registration process and then noticed the key was for room 13. Not that I'm superstitious, mind you, but I should have realized, given how the trip had gone up to that point, that the number thirteen augured poorly. But with a key finally in hand, I could not have been happier had the proprietor given me Will Rogers' favorite lariat. Only when departing the office did I spy a small sign placed low on the wall next to the exit that proclaimed dogs prohibited!

*Too late, evil dog haters! You'll have to rip this key from my turtled fist. Consider this cultural payback for my last overly spiced Indian curry that gave me the runs.*

I parked the car in an out-of-the-way spot. On opening the rear door for Dice to exit and after pushing aside some hanging clothing, I discovered a thoroughly chewed backseat and macerated armrest. At last the origin for the mysterious noises had become clear. I shook my head dejectedly. What other tricks could Dice possibly still have up his furry sleeve?

I leashed up Dice and furtively walked him behind the motel to do his business. Then I draped Dice with my dark jacket and hurried him through the door and into room 13. I was exhausted. Within minutes I had turned out the lights, piled into bed, pulled up the covers, and slipped into the waiting arms of Morpheus.

In the wee hours, menacing growling followed by ferocious barking caused me to stir. I was only semiconscious when an eighty-pound, sharp-clawed animal raced across my bed, raking my exposed skin. Dice's outburst jolted me to full alertness. I feared eviction for having broken the rule about having a dog in the room. Adrenaline gushed through my veins like water from a fire hydrant. Maintaining a warm bed during the wee hours suddenly became my paramount goal.

I leapt blindly from the bed, struck the corner of the dresser, cursed aloud, and hobbled toward my then totally out-of-control Dalmatian. On finally reaching him, with difficulty I held his jaws together and whispered, "Shut up, you moron, or you'll get us tossed out." After a few more minutes of muted growling, Dice finally calmed and became his usual friendly self. At last I returned to bed.

The following morning I prepared to begin a new day. Feeling optimistic after a night's rest, I emerged from the room scrubbed, flossed, and with Dice leashed for his morning walk and—*was busted*. To my dismay, not one but two police cruisers with radios squawking and blue lights blinking sat parked immediately in front of my room. I realized Oklahoma was no longer the Wild West, requiring federal marshals from Fort Smith, but sending two police cars for the niggling crime of stowing away a dog seemed an overreaction.

On spotting me, a ruddy-complexioned, shovel-nosed man in a deputy sheriff's uniform approached me. His belly spilled over his belt like ten pounds of potatoes from a five-pound bag. He pushed his hat back on his head, revealing his forehead had largely annexed his scalp.

"Good morning, officer," I said meekly, wondering if I should offer my wrists for cuffing or wait till asked.

"Mornin'," the officer said in his soft-spoken drawl. He sounded straight out of the cast of *Oklahoma*, but he soon dispensed with further social niceties. "You git robbed last night?" he drawled, the corners of his bushy eyebrows pointing toward his broad expanse of fleshy forehead.

It took a few beats for me to realize the deputy had not come to arrest me. I did a mental pirouette and began to scrutinize the contents of my billfold. I found the cash and credit cards intact. I then surveyed my room for missing valuables and in due course answered the officer in the negative.

"You sure now?" the lawman asked while shifting his considerable weight from one black boot to another. His dark eyes studied me quizzically.

"Sure am, Officer. Nothing missing."

"Strange," the deputy replied, rubbing the deep cleft in his chin with the back of his meaty hand. "Every one these here twelve rooms before you and the three on the other side got hit by a sneak thief last night. Picked 'em clean, he did. For some odd reason, this light-fingered thief just up and skipped your room. Now I just cain't figure why he would do such a thing?"

I, on the other hand, immediately could. The rescuer of my

billfold, credit cards, and other valuables was standing at my side with his usual walleyed appearance. Just then Dice gazed up at me with what seemed to me an expression of pure vindication. *I'll swear that dog's grinning. Way to go, Dicey Dog!*

Later that morning I drove west on Interstate 40 across Oklahoma and into the Texas panhandle. The open expanse of land had given rise to a feeling of hopefulness, perhaps like that experienced by the pioneers when first viewing the vastness of the prairies. Dice, too, had awakened, gazing at the largely uninhabited grasslands and the ribbon of highway stretching straight out before us. Of this flat land it was said your dog could leave home and you could still see him three days later.

At Amarillo I turned south onto Interstate 27 and headed across the Llano Estacado, or Staked Plains. Coronado and his fellow conquistadores had centuries before pounded stakes to navigate the featureless Llano to assure their return to New Spain. *What kind of people spring from this barren, table-flat land? What characteristics would this sparsely inhabited environment lend to the people who homesteaded here and whose offspring still reside here today?*

In the intervening three hundred fifty years, the scenery on the Llano Estacado had changed little, but now at least road signs marked the way. Dice rode quietly in the backseat with what I interpreted as a smug look plastered across his muzzle. Intermittently I heard vigorous ear flapping akin to the sound of a hovering helicopter. I reached back periodically to stroke his silky fur and received soft, wet licks in return.

I arrived in Lubbock just before the setting sun painted the western rim of sky brilliant shades of orange and red. Lubbock has the prettiest sunsets anywhere, and the local denizens disingenuously claim the view is unimpaired by compromising hills or trees.

In the morning the sun would ascend over Prairie Dog Town in Mackenzie Park and shine down on Ransom Canyon where once Spanish and Anglo traders negotiated with the Comanche for the return of hostages. The breaking day would also bring a new beginning for my family, in a novel place, where a fresh chapter in our lives would begin to unfold. The day would further impart a much-needed second (or eighty-eighth) chance for our inveterate malefactor, Dice.

I was feeling less stressed than I had at the outset of our journey. My muscles felt looser, my mind more expansive, and I felt more hopeful. Earlier worries about the new job and finding a suitable home now struck me as less daunting. Things would work out, I thought. How did I know we would experience such good fortune?

After all, I'd been lucky enough to avoid a sneak thief due to a very loyal, if not terribly bright Dalmatian. Surely, good luck, along with the incorrigible Dice, must have been riding shotgun with me.

And for better or worse, Houston, the Eagle has landed—and Dicey Dog is anxious to explore his new home.

## Chapter 8

# THE MAN WHO PLAYED PINOCHLE WITH DOGS

*We must admit that the divine banquet of the brain was, and still is, a feast with dishes that remain elusive in the blending, and with sauces whose ingredients are even now a secret.*

—MacDonald Critchley

*The brain gives the heart its sight. The heart gives the brain its vision.*

—Rob Kall

The paging system squawked my name, reminding me of my lateness for clinic. I glanced out the window and viewed a rust-colored crescent on the horizon. The boiling dust cloud seemed to enlarge by the moment. I felt a sense of dread, knowing Lubbock would soon be engulfed by the dust storm. I hurried toward the neurology clinic, feeling apprehensive, twice glancing out windows at the approaching storm.

As I drew near, I could see a packed waiting room. From a distance, the patients' chatter sounded like a flock of geese. As I approached, faces turned expectantly and the din diminished. Many of those in the waiting room wore denim jeans, cowboy hats, and cotton shirts or colorful, puffed-sleeve blouses. Others dressed in fashionable clothing or logo-bearing sportswear. I estimated fifty people in the waiting room—many with curious faces and trembling hands.

I switched my black bag to my right hand, nodded in what I hoped was a confident manner, and burst through the clinic door.

I must be nuts. Residents, interns, medical students, and several staff neurologists would work such large clinics back in Minnesota—never a job for a single neurologist!

I greeted the impatient-looking clinic nurses and strode toward an overflowing chart rack. The intake note read: "75-year-old farmer from Muleshoe, eight-year history of PD for med check." The message also listed his current medicines.

*Wasn't Muleshoe that cotton town northwest of Lubbock nearby the infamous Bloated Goat Saloon?* College friends had told me about this boot-scooting, brawl-provoking watering hole.

The chart's heft suggested the patient had attended the Tarbox clinic for years. Not long after the medical school had been established in 1969, the Texas legislature had established the Tarbox Parkinson's Disease Institute to honor a beloved Lubbock-area state representative who suffered with the disorder. Such benevolence had occurred frequently when Texas held vast reserves of oil that could be readily converted into revenues for pet legislative projects. In recent years, the flow of both oil and funding had stemmed. Even worse, the dean of the medical school had redirected much of the Tarbox funding to support cash-starved basic science departments. The Parkinson's disease cause had soldiered on with substantially reduced resources.

The faculty champion for Parkinson's disease, Doctor Joseph Bianchine, had in the meantime decamped for the security of a faculty position at the Ohio State School of Medicine. He still returned monthly to Lubbock to hold a clinic, but his visits had failed to keep pace with an increasing patient load. The gulf between patient needs and physician services had prompted the recruitment of a full-time faculty neurologist. In hindsight, the job description should have specified, "Must have experience with Parkinson's disease and *substantial quixotic leanings.*"

I scanned prior chart notes, planned my examination, and mentally considered my treatment options. Like battle plans at the onset of war, my considerations would soon become obsolete.

As I entered the room, an elderly man sitting upon the exam table glared at me. I noticed he was of small stature, with a face as fissured as a prune.

"What's keeping you, doc, out playing golf?"

*What a day to golf! Would have to nail my shoes to the tee box.*

"Sorry to keep you, Mr. Woodley. I'm Doctor Hutton. What can I do for you today?"

The man peered down his nose like a hawk sizing up its prey. He wore a mauve sweatshirt that screamed in bold letters, "If things get better with age, then I'm approaching MAGNIFICENCE." From beneath the bill of a dirty, pulled-down Dallas Cowboys cap, he scrutinized me through slit-like eyes. I slowly lowered myself onto the wheeled stool and tried to act nonchalant, as if I had ample time to wait out his petulance.

"It's nice to *finally* see you," he intoned, not yet willing to abandon his overwrought pique. "*Was* anxious to get to Muleshoe *before* the sandstorm hit." While his words were barbed, his western drawl and soft Parkinson's speech reduced their sting. Outside the wind began to wail, reaching just then the higher octaves. In unison our eyes went to the ceiling, as if making entreaties to an angry Mother Nature.

"Mr. Woodley, I see Doctor Bianchine has treated you."

I observed the corners of Sam Woodley's mouth turn up slightly. He nodded his head. He ran a gnarled old hand along the table, smoothing the hygienic paper.

"Yep, for years Doc Bianchine has been my doctor. Without him I'd be moving slower 'n a constipated slug. Liked that funny-talking Yankee, mind you, even if the son of a bitch rooted for the wrong team," Sam said, pointing up at his Dallas Cowboys cap.

I continued with my get-acquainted conversation, sensing a thaw in my frigid reception.

"So, watch sports, do you?"

"Do now. Wife up and died three years ago. My kid took off for godless California. Not much else to do since leasing out the farm."

After a few sympathetic clucks, I asked, "Live by yourself?"

"Yep, but, sonny, ya see a young heifer wantin' to play house with an old fart like me, ya let me know!" A mischievous grin came over his gnomish, weather-beaten face.

I felt myself beginning to admire the pluck of this old cotton farmer. "I'll keep it in mind, Mr. Woodley. How you spending your time these days?"

"Frankly, not doin' much. Try to care for the place as best I can. Played cards with my Gladys, before the cancer took her." Before he turned his head away, I noticed his eyes had begun to glisten. His defiance by then was melting faster than an ice cube on a Texas sidewalk in July. He then struck me as appearing vulnerable and painfully lonely.

Trying to avoid restoking his ire or further reducing him to tears, I steered the conversation toward the safer topic of his health.

"What problems are you having with your Parkinson's disease?"

In a muted voice, Sam began describing difficulty when cutting his food and tying his shoelaces. His tremor and shuffling feet embarrassed him. He surprised me by saying that he also found it harder now to shuffle cards.

*Shuffling cards? Why does he need to shuffle cards? Solitaire?*

In response to my questioning, Sam Woodley conceded that his memory had slipped a bit. I listened, nodded, and sympathized. We discussed making lists to jog his memory. I inquired about side effects of his medicine.

"Upset stomach or vomiting?"

"Nah, Doc. Cast-iron stomach."

I asked a further series of unproductive questions. Then I

asked a standard, almost throw-away question: "Have you ever seen animals or people that were not really there?"

He hesitated. I noticed his jaw muscles tighten. I sat motionless on my mobile stool, anticipating his response. His face took on a quizzical look that could not have appeared more puzzled had I hopped off my stool, stood on my head, and begun to spit out marbles. Sam measured me; his bushy eyebrows knitted up like two angry caterpillars about to do battle.

"Maybe, maybe not."

"Well, could you help me out a little bit more?"

He ran the back of his hand across his square chin. I observed his lips quiver ever so slightly. I felt Sam Woodley held a secret that he had not planned to share that day.

After taking an unusual interest in the ceiling tiles, Sam Woodley finally dropped his head and blurted out dryly, "Well, Doc, I see some dawgs."

At last, he had shared it. I quickly followed up. "Dogs, huh? Well, big or little dogs?" I asked in my best nonjudgmental tone but feeling my interest piqued.

Sam Woodley wrung leathery hands and tugged at a dangling earlobe. With a weary sigh, his resistance gave way like a tractor suddenly extracted from a mud hole. He then began to share his well-guarded mystery—and in so doing, related a bizarre and unforgettable story.

Sometimes patients allow doctors to gain a glimpse of their most intimate secrets. Such trust must be earned, as it resides at the core of the doctor-patient relationship. Sam Woodley allowed me a premature gift that day like an early Christmas present, an information bequest that provided me insight and a most challenging dilemma.

"Well, 'bout every afternoon three dawgs drop by the house." He fell silent, awaiting my response to this snippet.

"Go on," I gently urged.

In his monotone he proceeded to describe a large, yellow Labrador, a black-and-white border collie, and a smaller white-and-light-brown cocker spaniel.

"Are they scary?" I asked.

"Nah, gentle as can be; besides, we play together."

Puzzled and unsure where the conversation was leading, but wanting him to share more, I asked if the dogs had names.

He nodded. "I call them Yellow Dawg, the Lab; Skipper, the border collie; and Coco, the spaniel."

"Well, what do they do at your house?"

"Mostly like to play cards."

I wondered if my ears were tricking me. "Oh, I see," I replied, trying to sound collected, as if I often heard of dogs playing cards. "Well, what card games do y'all play?"

"Usually pinochle, their favorite."

"So, play pinochle, do they?"

"Oh, yeah, especially Skipper and Coco."

"I see. . . . Make any noise while they play?"

"Nope, never a sound, but I know what they want."

"Well, Mr. Woodley, please tell me how you and the dogs go about playing pinochle."

Sam Woodley proceeded to describe how he would place the card table in a certain configuration and arrange the dogs' favorite chairs. He would invite the dogs to jump onto their chairs and begin the game.

"Coco really likes to beat the boys. Makes her damned upset if she loses; been known to leave in a big huff."

He related how he would shuffle and deal the cards but of late had been having difficulty managing the cards. Nevertheless, he went on to say that his canine friends had even greater difficulty than he, forcing him to always shuffle and deal.

"You see, Doc, my hands don't shuffle as good as before this here Mr. Parkinson's disease. Be obliged if you'd just, well, give it back to him!" With his quip, an endearing smile spread across his weathered, old face.

"Maybe I can help," I encouraged. Intrigued by his narrative, I nodded for him to continue.

"Well, Skipper, the border collie, wears these here green eye shades—you know, like bookkeeper types wear—and, uh . . .Coco, the cocker spaniel, sits on a pink silk handkerchief while she plays. Thinks it makes her lucky. Oh, and Coco sits with the floorboards, not across them. Feels real strong 'bout this, just like my Gladys did. Guess both were a might superstitious. Suspect Yellow Dawg comes mostly for the sandwiches; great appetite, not so good at pinochle. Yellow Dawg has a good time, though. Generally's got a big ole smile across his muzzle."

My mind was reeling, visualizing this elaborate scene. I concentrated, trying not to project incredulity.

Sam Woodley was relating an unreal event with the same nonchalance as if he were explaining the weather conditions or the state of the region's cotton crop. Could his elaborate hallucination have been prompted by Cassius Marcellus Coolidge's series of pictures, *Dogs Playing Poker*? My knowledge of pinochle was far from extensive, but I knew it was a game for two to four people and not a pastime for visiting dogs.

In my mind, I had already determined that Sam Woodley's medicine would have to be changed to rid him of his hallucinations. I foresaw no other option.

With twinkling brown eyes under his bushy eyebrows, Sam warmed to his narrative and became still more animated. I observed his hand tremor increase. He described his daily visitation in unmistakably affectionate and enthusiastic tones.

"I always make sandwiches before they come. Yellow Dawg likes ham and cheese and lots of 'em; the spaniel and collie prefer turkey but hold the lettuce."

He related how he also prepared snacks consisting of chips and dog biscuits.

"They prefer the beef-flavored biscuits."

I sensed Sam took pride in his role as host and spent considerable time preparing for his visitors.

"I put down a bowl of water—just in case they get a might thirsty."

"Mr. Woodley, can you reach out and touch the dogs?"

"Nah, funny you mention that. If I try and pat them, my hand passes right through 'em like they're ghosts. Makes 'em disappear. A long time ago learned not to try it."

"What about smelling the dogs?"

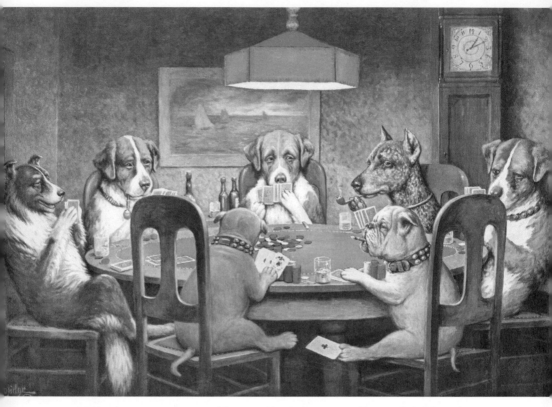

Might this painting, *A Friend in Need* by Cassius Marcellus Coolidge, have been a model for Sam Woodley's elaborate hallucinations of dogs playing pinochle? (Courtesy of DiMarco Productions, Las Vegas, NV)

"You know, hadn't thought 'bout it, but can't smell 'em, feel 'em, or hear 'em neither."

I paused and considered for a few moments just what he had related. Sam Woodley's hallucinations were visual, lacking sound, smell, or touch. The hallucinations were vivid and occurred day after day and disappeared if he tried to touch them. His description fit well the medicine-related side effects of Parkinson's disease but was more complex than I had previously encountered.

"When we're fixin' to finish the game, dawgs jump down and head for the door. Don't know where they live but well

cared for. Plum happy to see me, they are. Just disappear without me even opening up the door."

"Do you and the dogs play anything besides cards?" I was
curious to learn the extent of his interaction with his illusory
dogs and his emotional dependence on them.

Sam thought for a minute before replying. "Watch the Cowboys on TV. Don't know about America's team, but sure as hell
are the dawgs' favorite." Sam laughed heartily. With his laughter, his hand tremor again increased in amplitude, acting like
his emotional barometer.

"How do you know that?"

"Well, Cowboys make 'em a touchdown, Skipper jumps off
the couch and tears around the room, jumping over furniture—
his own little end-zone celebration, it is. If other team scores,
dawgs lay chins on their paws, look real sad, and pout awhile.
Pretty easy to read my dawgs."

As Mr. Woodley spoke, I was becoming even more certain
that his hallucinations needed to be stopped. I inhaled deeply
and began to interpret his current symptoms and how I thought
I could improve his treatment.

"Mr. Woodley, a healthy person's ability to move about is
like a wagon normally pulled by a team of eight horses. With
Parkinson's, only two healthy horses remain to haul the wagon.
To keep it moving, we must urge the horses harder with medicines—much like swinging a whip over the horses' heads."

Sam Woodley sat quietly, listening to my analogy, one I
hoped this rural dweller could relate to.

"Unfortunately, whipping the horses too hard can cause
them to get balky or in your case cause side effects, such as seeing things not really there."

Sam Woodley received my words without comment or
change in facial expression but did intermittently nod his head.
I continued by explaining how Parkinson's disease had diminished his brain's store of dopamine and that his levodopa/car-
bidopa medicine supplemented his brain's inadequate supply
of dopamine.

"You see, Mr. Woodley, too much treatment causes a spill-over effect, causing visual hallucinations. Mr. Woodley, we must reduce your medicine."

Sam Woodley sat motionless for a long time. Then his mouth began to make chewing movements, as if he first had to chew his thoughts into declarative sentences. His expression was pensive. He wrapped his arms across his chest.

I plowed on, assuring him that by reducing his medicine, we could banish his hallucinatory hounds. I added a small disclaimer that we might encounter some worsening in his movement and then paused for his questions.

Sam Woodley replied simply, "Don't know 'bout that, Doc."

I was taken aback. "Well, Mr. Woodley, don't you agree that we need to get rid of your hallucinations?"

"Well, Doc, dawgs ain't bothering me none."

I considered what further arguments might be made. "Are you worried about your movements worsening?"

"Nah, not a worry, got plenty of time to get my dab of work done." Sam Woodley chewed a little more before finally asking, "But how would I spend my afternoons, if I didn't play pinochle with my friends?"

His question left me speechless. For long moments I thought how best to proceed. Finally I blurted, "But don't you want to stop your hallucinations?"

"Well, I'd damn sure miss my dawg friends! I know that."

I searched my memory for a medical bon mot, but before finding one, Sam Woodley added, "Besides, Doc, whatever would I do with all the extra sandwiches?"

Such rarified moments of absolute irrationality provide insight. Certainly I gained that day a better understanding of Sam Woodley's unmet emotional needs. But the experience also had taught me to spend more effort viewing the situation through the other person's eyes, a valuable lesson both for the practice of medicine and in life in general. Whatever center in my brain had responsibility for listening—really listening to what patients' implied and not just what they said—shifted up a gear that day.

I had been trained throughout my specialization that hallucinations required adjustment of medicine. I knew hallucinations were often well tolerated, and even rarely, as with Sam Woodley, welcomed. However, I also knew that progression could occur and hallucinations could become frightening.

But as best I could determine, Sam Woodley showed no signs of any lurking hostility or incipient paranoia. He also claimed reduced boredom resulted from his hallucinations. My ambivalence raged. But still these hallucinations were florid and well developed. And what would my new colleagues think if they learned I had failed to address them?

Hours later, after having seen my final patient of the day, having completed my charting, and having shrunk a formidable stack of paperwork, I directed my fatigued footsteps toward the doctors' parking lot.

With great effort I pushed open the exterior door of the hospital and bent into a ferocious, paint-eating dust storm. I clutched my black bag near my chest and bent low to cross the parking lot to my car. Once there, I forced open the car door and quickly slipped in.

I sat there, catching my breath and scraping dirt from eyes, nose, and mouth. As my breathing slowed, my thoughts returned to my wizened patient, Sam Woodley. I hoped he had reached his home safely through the howling dust storm. I smiled, remembering his pugnacious approach to life.

I wondered, had his independent-mindedness arisen from a lifetime of farming cotton in borderline soil, violent weather, and semiarid conditions? Having always irrigated his cotton, was not Sam Woodley's shuttered life now in need of irrigation for his downcast spirits?

Sam Woodley's lack of human connectedness struck me as bleak as the flat, treeless topography on which he lived. The haunting barrenness of the Llano Estacado along with his loneliness, in concert with his medicine, had somehow given rise to his remarkable but illusory dogs.

I believed both internal and external factors contributed to his elaborate phantasm. One thing seemed certain. His dogs had provided him with an unusual form of companionship that had reduced his feelings of utter aloneness.

I felt a sense of satisfaction, knowing I had passed his inspection and gained sufficient trust for him to share his guarded secret. Thirty years later, I appreciate his trust no less.

I visualized Sam Woodley arriving at his remote farmhouse. Sam would have hurried into the house as fast as his shuffling gait would allow and set about arranging the card table. I imagined him carefully placing the table parallel to the floorboards and arranging the dogs' favorite chairs. Hopefully he had arrived with enough time to fix ham sandwiches in a quantity satisfactory to the Labrador and turkey sandwiches for his border collie and cocker spaniel. I imagined him placing bowls of dog biscuits and chips on the card table and a water bowl on the floor.

I felt a gritty smile cross my face, recalling my medical decision regarding his hallucinations. But I was confident that I had made the correct choice. At least it felt right to me, considering the nature of this highly individualistic man and his secluded lifestyle.

For now Sam Woodley would continue to enjoy his extraordinary pinochle parties with "his dawgs."

## Chapter 9

# AT THE FURROW'S END

*Babylon in all its desolation is a sight not so awful*

*As that of the human mind in ruins.*

—Scrope Berdmore Davies

Heavy double doors banged shut behind me. Like a jolt of electricity, anxiety surged through my body. I quickly located bed 21 and the unidentified woman who was responsible for my stat page to the medical intensive care unit. I placed my black bag on the small table alongside her hospital bed. A quick glance at the bed revealed a small body virtually eclipsed by monitors, a wheezing ventilator, and a virtual spaghetti bowl of wires and catheters.

I hastily scanned the labels of the intravenous bottles that hung at her bedside. The nearby table displayed printouts of her abnormal vital signs. All revealed worrisome numbers, causing me still greater apprehension.

Somewhere across the intensive care unit, a ventilator alarm shrieked, a telephone jingled, and infusion pumps thrummed. Nurses with intent facial expressions scurried about the unit on rubber-soled shoes, providing care for these, the very sickest of the hospital's sick.

It was late evening in March of 1995. I was the neurologist on call for the hospital. Unseasonable sleet was falling outside, as if Mother Nature had not quite finished punishing the denizens of the Texas South Plains. I was barely aware of the inclement weather, however, as by then my mind had focused on my task at hand. Already I had dismissed thoughts of my wife's home-cooked meal and of proud recitations by my children of their school activities.

I paged through the painfully thin hospital chart that lay on the bedside table. The "unknown woman" had collapsed in a large Lubbock discount store. An ambulance had been summoned, and she had been transported by EMS to the emergency room. The chart provided no additional information about the unfortunate patient.

I hurriedly examined her. Her left arm and leg were as limp as a Raggedy Ann doll. They were paralyzed. I called loudly to her. "Please open your eyes." She made no response. "Squeeze my fingers," I pleaded. I felt no contraction of her thin, cool, arthritic fingers. Ominously, her right pupil was enlarged ("blown," in the medical vernacular), and failed to constrict to the light from a strong flashlight. I thought if the eye is the window to the soul, then this portal had been tightly shuttered, with her awareness sucked deep into the black abyss of coma.

Her tiny body appeared to weigh less than eighty-five pounds. She seemed childlike and swallowed up by the large mechanical bed. The woman's hooked nose dominated other facial features, and her thin hair bore an unhealthy yellowish tinge. Sallow skin showed deep, craggy wrinkles much like the bark of an ancient olive tree. I was certain of one thing; time had been most unkind to this old woman.

Dirt beneath fingernails, arthritic knuckles, callused hands, and leathery skin suggested she had led an outdoor, physical existence. I wondered what labor this woman had performed to bring about such physical changes.

I located a folder of her X-rays. The film showing her head CT scan screamed out a dire message. A large blood clot lay buried within her right hemisphere, looking like a coiled serpent. The sanguineous, snakelike figure had shoved her brain violently leftward into her pitiless and unforgiving skull and looked likely to expand still further over the coming days. If that happened, it would crush the vital centers necessary for life itself.

After completing my examination and review of lab and X-ray studies, I wrote medical orders, dictated my consultation, and prescribed a drug that would combat the brain swelling that was sure to come. The deep location of the blood clot made it inaccessible to a scalpel, preventing a surgical option. Her moribund condition and our limited possibilities for treatment left me thoroughly disheartened. My earlier adrenaline rush slowly ebbed away. I sighed heavily and stood for several minutes, searching my mind for other treatment options that because of fatigue might have escaped me.

Finally, I turned to leave, but my pace was less hurried than it was on arrival. An astringent smell filled my nostrils. The incessant beeps and whirs of the equipment soon faded behind me as I departed the unit. I was mindful that the unknown woman's chance of surviving the night was poor.

To my surprise, the next morning I found her still clinging tenaciously to life. While her examination had improved minimally, she remained deeply comatose and gravely ill. I noticed a name had been posted at the end of her bed, a name that in this narrative we shall call Maggie Croft.

New laboratory and X-ray studies awaited my review. I was engrossed in ventilator settings, fluid input, bodily outputs, and other vital statistics, pondering additional ways to reduce her brain swelling, when from the corner of my eye I noticed an elderly man with hesitant, mincing steps approach the bedside. He was stooped, lean, and angular. His clothes looked frayed and fit him poorly. His dirty work boots likely had never seen a coat of polish, and his gray hair smacked of being home cut.

The man introduced himself as Ned Croft, husband of the patient. He sheepishly extended a callused, dirty hand. Mr. Croft avoided making eye contact. I sensed he was intimidated by the intensive care unit—a not unreasonable emotion given the strangeness of the surroundings. I suspected he had not previously experienced much contact with doctors or hospitals. I could only imagine his profound emotional shock at seeing his wife lying pale, motionless, and cradled within the massive mechanical bed.

I attempted to ease his tension by making sympathetic comments and by providing an update on his wife's condition. When he had relaxed somewhat, I explained the odds were sadly against her surviving such a massive stroke, but that a degree of hope still existed. His limited flow of words then halted, as surely as would a ship when sailing onto a rocky reef. He seemed lost for several minutes and deep within his own thoughts.

"Will you share your feelings with me, Mr. Croft?" I finally asked. I believed his venting would benefit him and might elicit helpful medical information. Unfortunately, he could not provide such a narrative, so I began to ask him specific questions.

"How long have you and Mrs. Croft been married?"

After a pause he appeared to gather himself. "Maggie 'n me married over sixty years." His words flowed out slowly like honey from a jar.

"Do you and Mrs. Croft have any children?"

"Never had children, just each other."

"What type of work have you and Mrs. Croft done?"

Ned briefly focused his attention on me for the first time and straightened his posture. "Maggie and me worked hard, powerful hard. Back in the Depression, times were bad. Followed the crops—picked cherries in New Mexico, but mostly cotton 'cross Texas."

"And how was Mrs. Croft as a cotton picker?"

"Never seen a cotton picker like my Maggie. Picked like she was fighting fire, she did," pronouncing *fire* as "far."

"She must have been really good at picking cotton." I had glimpsed a spark of passion in Mr. Croft and wished to fan it further into a flame.

"Land O' mighty, she was. At the end of the day, her hands be bleeding from the hulls, but her tow sack be fuller than t'other pickers."

The weathered face of Ned Croft began to radiate pride. Mr. Croft's gaze moved far away and a slight smile crossed his face. He appeared to be remembering those happier days from so long ago. Despite feeling the pressure of time and my other responsibilities, I was slow to draw Ned Croft back to the unwelcome present.

Finally, I again initiated the conversation. "And how did you and Mrs. Croft meet?"

"Both came from picker families. Met as kids, at the end of a long row of cotton. After a quick lesson back then, parents just left 'em there, hoping kids would learn to pick while they went on 'bout their own work. Us kids had to earn something—that cotton was good money."

"Did you and Maggie go to school?"

"Picked up a bit here and there. Mostly followed the crops; interfered with regular learning. In school for a month or two then on to the next place."

"And where did y'all get married?"

"Well," Ned said, shuffling his feet in place. "We never got married in no church or by a JP or nothing, but felt just as married. Wouldn't let no foreman separate me from my Maggie. They tried; wouldn't do it. Sometimes needed only one picker in a field and sent t'others off to another farmer's place. Lost some good work 'cause of it. Kind of felt like I needed to look out for my Maggie, and she said she sure 'nuf needed to look out for her Ned." Mr. Croft chuckled, recalling this tender interlude with obvious pleasure.

"Sounds like the work was hard."

"That's for sure. Wore out our backs bending over all day. Knees and hands got terrible tired."

Ned shared how he and Maggie had always been poor, still averting his eyes away from my face. "Maggie never had no fine dresses or other finery a'tall. But had one thing she really liked." Ned's voice grew in force and confidence as he spoke.

"What was that?"

"Saved my cash money, I did, and bought her a shiny locket. Gave it to her—kind of like a wedding present. Maggie near never took that locket off in sixty years."

After letting his touching words sink in, I then proceeded to obtain some necessary medical information from Mr. Croft. At the conclusion of our visit, he edged closer to the bedside. His wrinkled old hand grasped his wife's motionless one, a hand once so adept at separating the cotton from the hull. I saw Ned slip a silvery object into Maggie's fingers. He gently stroked Maggie's stringy hair away from her weathered face. I overhead him say, "Maggie, you left for the store in an awful big hurry. Forgot your locket."

He then made eye contact with me and straightened himself up to his full height of about six feet. In a quaking voice he pleaded, "Doc, do everything you can." His voice cracked and faltered before struggling on. He finally blurted out, "I . . . I love that old gal."

Those phrases, "I love that old gal" and "she picked cotton like she was fighting fire," echoed persistently through my mind. *Echoed* does not adequately describe my remembrance—as Ned Croft's words would haunt me for years.

After Ned's poignant description of his wife, I no longer could think of Maggie Croft as a shriveled old woman with failing physiology. She instead had become an energetic and skillful harvester who had been much loved by Ned. Maggie Croft had struggled through desperate decades tightly bonded to her husband. She had evoked the strongest display of public emotion of which I felt Ned Croft capable.

And struggle to save her life we did. The doctors and nurses labored tirelessly. The hospital staff would surround her bed, probing and checking, infusing and pondering. We addressed her brain swelling by dehydrating her brain and reducing carbon dioxide in her bloodstream; both efforts designed to eke out precious millimeters of space within her skull to buy time for the swelling and blood clot to recede. We balanced complicated bodily chemistry and addressed her fluid and nutritional needs. These treatments monopolized our time and distracted us from the near futility of our efforts. We tried every management strategy known to us in our dogged attempt to salvage the life of Maggie Croft—but in the end our efforts came to naught.

The following day, the dam of life gave way for Maggie. Her bodily systems began to fail, for which no reasonable or adequate therapy existed. Her vital signs and neurological functioning worsened inexorably. In the face of the massive insult to her brain, her body simply could no longer sustain the essence of life. Maggie Croft died with her husband blanketed over the bed rails, hovering protectively over her small, frail body. Ned's glistening brown eyes belied his outward stoicism.

After a time, I pronounced Maggie dead. Then I turned and embraced Ned Croft. Through his worn clothing, I felt his bony, sinewy body. In an almost courtly fashion, he straightened to his full height, took a step back, and thanked me repeatedly for my efforts with his simple but powerful words. I offered my heartfelt condolences to him. As if tethered, Ned stood alongside the sheet-draped, lifeless body of his wife, appearing uncertain as to what he should do next.

At last I saw Ned reach under the sheet and slip from Maggie's hand an old, tarnished, heart-shaped locket. At once I recognized the locket as her most prized possession, the one that Ned Croft had bought for her so many years and countless furrows before.

Mr. Croft seemed aware the time had come to leave the bedside, but he remained immobile, as if entangled like a fly in a spider's web in his own grief and uncertainty. Eventually with increased stooping and the locket dangling down from his hand, Ned shuffled toward the exit of the intensive care unit. A silvery glint flashed from the locket when he passed beneath a ceiling light. I saw him draw in the locket and place it near his heart in the breast pocket of his work shirt. Ned Croft appeared as lost and bewildered as anyone I had ever encountered.

I wondered if Ned Croft, after spending his life with Maggie, knew which part of his existence belonged to him and which part was a combination of the two of them. I imagined when Mr. Croft eventually left Lubbock alone, it would be the first time in sixty years when he would pack his own few possessions. Would he learn to prepare his meals? Who would massage his tired, sore back at the end of a long day of harvesting? I felt deeply saddened both for Maggie Croft's death and for her partner's lonely plight.

Over the years, I have reflected on Ned and Maggie Croft's strong love for one another. I have wondered how their bond survived undiminished for so many years. Their affection was evident but certainly seemed not based on physical beauty. Neither Maggie nor Ned, at least at their advanced age, could have been described in appearance as anything but plain.

Maggie and Ned had proved unsuccessful by the materialistic measures of our society. They had never earned sufficient money to amass many possessions, a comfortable lifestyle having always eluded them. I imagined that supervisors had dealt with them and other migrant laborers little different from how foremen generations earlier had dealt with slaves; their lives were never valued for much more than the amount of crops they picked. I knew that Maggie and Ned had lived a vagabond existence, traveling in search of crops to harvest. Based on my experience with them, neither had benefited from formal education nor held any deep understanding of music, art, or philosophy. Little time would have been available in their work-filled days to reflect on the meaning of their existence or the metaphysical nature of their relationship. They had produced no children who might have further bonded their relationship or added enriching texture to their lives. Yet there they were, a pair of octogenarians with an unbreakable union forged through mutual struggle, constant companionship, and a durable love.

Their relationship had fully watered the soil of their existence. The seeds of their relationship sprang forth, resisting their many cruel adversities.

I have often recalled Ned Croft's slow pace as he departed the intensive care unit that day. Ned initially pushed at the swinging doors, opening them just a crack. He then glanced back at his deceased wife's body, his eyes vacant and wanting. I saw a tear stream down his aged face. By then in common with him both the nurse and I had tear-stained cheeks.

My final impression of Ned was of a mournful old man, struggling to regain his emotional footing, his equilibrium as disrupted as a hummingbird in a windstorm. Ned Croft with his tattered appearance and pained emotions abruptly was lost from view as the doors slammed shut behind him.

The complexity of love has baffled the wisest sages. Poets and lyricists have written extensively and eloquently. But for me, Ned's simple utterance said it best. "Doc, I love that old gal."

## Chapter 10
# PINOCHLE REDUX

*Shaped a little like a loaf of French country bread,*

*Our brain is a crowded chemistry lab,*

*Bustling with nonstop neural conversations.*

—Diane Ackerman

*Without the mind sensuality quite has no organs to call her own!*

—J. D. Salinger

One of the most dramatic medical breakthroughs of the twentieth century occurred with the discovery of L-dopa for the treatment of Parkinson's disease. I loved the 1990 movie *Awakening* based on the book by Oliver Sacks and starring Robin Williams, Robert De Niro, and Julie Kavner. It nicely illustrated the phenomenal improvement from L-dopa in persons suffering from postencephalitic parkinsonism. The movie also sadly demonstrated how over time the L-dopa response shortened and serious side effects developed.

Not long after the advent of L-dopa, researchers began searching for newer medicines that would stimulate the same brain sites as L-dopa, but would result in longer-lasting benefits with fewer side effects. This new class of drugs became known as dopamine agonists. Like L-dopa, these L-dopa impersonators have two roles. Not only do they benefit bodily movement, but they also mediate the rewards system, guiding people toward food, drink, mates, and other areas necessary for human survival. Tinkering with the dopamine system risks altering this unique rewards system and may result in unwanted outcomes such as compulsive gambling, overeating, drug addiction, and hypersexuality.

The following story emerged from a clinical trial of one of these experimental agonists and tells of its strange impact on the lives of two unique people.

Cotton strippers had already denuded millions of the stubby plants of their short staple fiber on the South Plains of Texas—the largest inland cotton-producing area in the United States. Gins hummed twenty-four hours a day, seven days a week, belching out gray plumes of dust and lint while refining the soft, white determinant of either success or failure for the local economy.

On Friday nights colorfully dressed partisans filled high school football stadiums, and on Saturdays face-painted fraternity guys, pretty coeds, and other assorted black-and-red-garbed Red Raider fans packed the tradition-filled Jones Stadium at Texas Tech University (known as Jones AT&T Stadium as of 2000). That fall in 1982, life on the Llano Estacado had a feeling of predictability, familiarity, and normalcy. However, such feelings of certainty and inevitability escaped a select few.

The soft western drawl of Sam Woodley reached my ear even before I entered the exam room. I passed Cheryl as she exited, handing me a slip of paper as she passed. I only glanced at her nurse's note before fixing my gaze on Sam Woodley. It had been more than a year since I had felt pressed by clinical circumstances to adjust his Parkinson's disease medicines, effectively banishing his hallucinated dogs. My decision had been prompted at the time by an addition to the pack of a large, mean-looking dog that had upset Sam.

Sam's gnomish figure sat perched on the blue vinyl examination table, his deeply fissured face cast downward. I noted he wore khaki slacks and a dress shirt with a button-down collar. *Uncharacteristic clothing for this Muleshoe farmer.*

"Well, Sam, you've had a birthday since your last visit. Happy birthday." I always began clinic visits with light banter, finding it enjoyable and surprisingly informative.

"Yup, officially just got older than dirt."

"How're things around Muleshoe?"

"Drier 'n moon dust—least 'twas last time I was there." He said this with a low level of peevishness but less than his customary roiling passion. I enjoyed and had come to expect his usual clinic exhortations; however, I felt just then like a fisherman whose bait the bass refused to take.

"Thought you lived on the farm?"

"Spending more 'n half my time smack dab here in Lubbock—hub of the great South Plains." Sam lifted his eyes in mock awe.

"Why you spending so much time in Lubbock?"

"With a friend," he chuckled and then paused. Sam stroked his clean-shaven face, carried out a few chewing movements, and chose his words carefully: "Mostly shopping the malls, eating itty-bitty French pastries, and slugging down troughs of herbal tea."

*Is this the same Sam Woodley I know?* I recalled his typical plucky defiance, braggadocio, and lack of political correctness. I now sensed him changed—more cowed, as well as surprisingly duded up for a country boy.

"Sam, you seem different. Is it because you're still missing those dogs of yours?"

"Missed 'em dawgs sure 'nuf for a piece, especially Skipper, the border, and Coco, the cocker. Yellow Dog was eating me out of house, farm, and chicken shack. Miss him less than a skunk with an attitude—saving *mucho* bucks on sandwich fixin's. Sure don't miss that mean cur of a dog. Pined for those card games for a spell, I did. Now I know'd those hounds were all in my head, but sure seemed real enough. Strange thing a mind—can play funny tricks on an *hombre*."

"You feeling lonesome without your dogs?"

"Nah, not so much now. I got me some human company now. Has advantages, know what I mean?"

I failed to grasp the implication and did not press the point further. I completed my examination and adjusted his Parkinson's medicines. As I wrote my chart note, I looked closer at Cheryl's note. She had written that Sam Woodley seemed less verbally combative and more withdrawn. She had scrawled in the margin "Poss. Depression."

As Sam and I chatted, it struck me that he was not wearing his favorite sweatshirt that claimed in bold letters if things improved with age then he must be approaching MAGNIFICENCE. Nor was he wearing his ever-present, grimy Dallas Cowboys cap. He had even shockingly replaced dirty work boots with tasseled brown loafers. Sam still expressed a degree of orneriness, to be sure, but he acted more subdued, almost placid, most un-Sam-like, I thought. He did not appear depressed, only calmer. I mentally shrugged it off, attributing it to his having a bad day or fatigue. Besides, being thirty minutes behind in clinic spurred me to cut corners and move along.

About an hour later, I passed behind the check-in desk and peered into the waiting area for the Tarbox Parkinson's disease clinic. There I glimpsed Sam Woodley with his crossed leg displaying his stylish tasseled loafer. *Why's he still hanging around the clinic?*

I returned to my work, burning through four or five patients at record pace, trying to get back on schedule. The next chart was that of a Mary Rose Sorenson, a woman of deep southern extraction who because of her husband's petroleum-related employment had landed in West Texas. After his untimely death, Mary Rose's opinion of Lubbock proved sufficiently to her liking to remain. Wags in the Parkinson's disease support group had claimed Homer Sorenson's fatal automobile accident might have been his only escape from Mary Rose's incessant nagging.

"Well, Mary Rose, how are you today?" I said on entering the examination room.

Whenever possible Mary Rose refused the nurse's request to change into the open-backed "see more" exam gown, though it would seem that day not for reasons of modesty.

Mary Rose was sixty years old and wore skin-tight blue jeans, a revealing, low-cut, leopard-print blouse with decorative spray of sequins, and knee-high red boots with four-inch heels. Her dyed-blond hair was loosely coiffed. While Mary Rose had always behaved in a genteel fashion around me, she still struck me as having a small iron fist hidden within a fashionable glove.

She had volunteered for a clinical research trial of a new treatment for her Parkinson's disease and had proved reliable, an accurate reporter of symptoms, and a constant irritant to my nurses.

"Oh, Doctor Hutton, ah feel so much better on this new medicine," Mary Rose said in her lilting southern accent.

"Mary Rose, you're looking better, even younger."

"Yes, I'm sure 'nuf feeling younger too."

I began filling out the various research forms but continued the light banter. Several times her conversation drifted to personal aspects of her life that carried faint but unmistakable sexual overtones. Male doctors become attuned to potentially provocative female patients and develop guarded instincts. Nevertheless, Mary Rose did not strike me so much as flirting as enjoying her role as a coquette.

"Well, Mary Rose, have you developed any side effects on this new medicine?"

"These sweet little pills brought about certain, shall we say, changes in me."

"What kind of changes?" I said, reaching for the adverse event form.

"Well, bless your heart, Doctor, I've been feeling like I'm twenty-one all over again. Feeling interested in men folk again. It's been such a long time." As she said this she ran her hands over her jean-clad thighs.

"So you're wanting male companionship?"

"Well, darling, desiring more than their companionship." She gazed downward with a demure look on her face.

"Do I understand you're having feelings of a sexual nature?"

"Surely as there's hospitality in old Charleston town," Mary Rose said, coyly again dropping her head, as if blushing.

"Well, Mary Rose, didn't know you even had a boyfriend, since your husband died, now how long ago was that?"

"Five years ago Homer passed."

"When did this upsurge of interest begin?"

"Very first day of the new pills. It's like my tank was empty but these pills just filled it plumb up."

"Does this concern you?"

"Not a bit. It's wonderful actually," she said, laughing. "Give me a box of these here Cupid pills and I'll sell them with my own personal testimony at the South Plains Mall. No, not a concern for little ole Mary Rose."

"What is your concern then?"

"Well, you remember Sam Woodley?"

"Of course, he was in here earlier."

"Well, he and I—sort of an item—last several months."

"That's great, glad you and Sam have become friends. So what's the problem?"

"Well, actually we're more than just friends. Met him at a support group meeting. Frankly didn't think much of him at first—you know the rough-hewn type, all countrified, dirty, and smelling like machinery. Lately, though, have found him more appealing in some ways, you might say, than my girlfriends. We were both lonesome and began to travel back and forth a lot. Trips plumb wore us out. Began spending time at each other's houses. Mercy me, if my girlfriends back in Charleston could see me now, wallowing in sin like a mockingbird in a birdbath."

Mary Rose announced this with a playful look on her flawlessly made-up face.

"Mary Rose, is there something you want to ask me?"

"Doctor, there's, uh, this problem."

"What's your problem?"

"Well, I don't have the problem. Sam has the problem."

"What? I don't quite follow."

"You see, Sam needs something for, for his manliness." Her quaint phrasing and pleading look were compelling.

"What exactly do you mean?"

"His organ needs tuning, so to speak." She displayed a limp wrist.

"Are you saying Sam's having trouble getting an erection?"

"Exactly, you've hit the nail smack dab on its head." Mary Rose now had risen to the task of fully explaining her concerns. "Sam's been tailing off on me like a castrated bull. Let me go get him, he's just out in the waiting room." Before I could begin to respond, Mary Rose had jumped from her chair and raced out of the exam room. She returned shortly with a sheepish Sam Woodley in tow. She pulled Sam into the room with a firm grasp on his starched collar.

"Howdy, long time no see," Sam said, obviously embarrassed by his summoning.

"Now, Sam, you go ahead and tell the doctor your big problem, or should we say your small problem. Now go on, he hasn't got all day."

"Well, you know, Doc, how I was feeling lonely and all, and well, Mary Rose and I, were kind of drawn to each other. One of your talks was where we met." Sam paused and appeared flummoxed as to how to proceed further. His mouth began making chewing movements. His eyes kept darting over to where Mary Rose sat.

"Sam, would you be more comfortable discussing this without Mary Rose present."

He nodded his head. "Some things kinda personal," he drawled.

I asked a newly petulant Mary Rose if she would mind waiting a few minutes at the nurse's workstation, knowing that for fobbing her off on them, the nurses would later harass me like a communist at a John Birch Society meeting.

"Now, Sam, what's going on with you?"

"Remember me telling how I was hurting pretty bad for female company?"

"Remember it well."

"Doc, trust me, I like getting it on as good as anyone, more than most. Had been ten long years since I'd been with a woman. Can get real far behind in ten years, but sure 'nuf after meeting Mary Rose, I got caught up real fast."

"Well, what's the problem then?"

"Never heard of a woman liked doing it as much as Mary Rose. Doc, she wants it three, four times a day. Tried to hang with her for a few days, making excuses like needing to visit the feed store or the barbershop. Could only get so many haircuts before I flat ran outta hair, and my barn is done stuffed full of feed. And with her always waiting back at the house in her red, see-through nightgown, wiggling her finger at me like a damned hooker and wantin' me to follow her down the hallway. Well, Doc, that woman's insatiable—damn nympho, you ask me."

"I'm getting the picture."

"Mary Rose's been ragging on me being impotent. Says I'm only half a man. Says she can't figure me out. Demands I buy some strong medicine to get me back in the game. Hell, Doc, I'm worn to a frazzle. My pecker's done pooped out."

"Thanks for sharing with me, Sam. I think I can help. By any chance does all this relate to the change in the way you're dressing?"

"Had to do something to get free of the house. Spent hours with her at St. Clair's department store in Muleshoe perusing fancy duds. How many times can you go through the same racks of clothes? Same thing in Lubbock, mostly at Hemphill's; became quite the shopper I did. Drug it out best I could. She hated the way I dressed, so this satisfied another of the changes she wanted for old Sambo. I took to doing anything she wanted, so long as it didn't take me anywhere near the bedroom."

I knew Sam Woodley was in his seventies. It was unreasonable to expect him to perform at anywhere near the pace demanded by Mary Rose. But what about Mary Rose? She was no spring chicken herself.

A few minutes later I asked Mary Rose to come back into the exam room. Behind her in the hallway, I saw Cheryl telegraph me a dirty look.

"Mary Rose, Sam shared his story. Puts a little different slant on it."

"He just needs medicine to put the lead back in his pencil, that's all."

"Well, Mary Rose, Sam says your libido is really high. Says you want sex three or four times a day."

"Not denying it, but I expect him to keep up. He's the Texas cowboy."

Sam sat glumly in the corner, looking about as happy as if he were being paraded down University Avenue stark naked.

"Let me see if I can explain what is going on here." I looked intently at Mary Rose and Sam before launching into my explanation. "We have encountered an unusual side effect from this new medicine Mary Rose is taking. Actually, many medicines for Parkinson's disease have, on very rare occasions, caused hypersexuality. The medicines stimulate the brain's dopamine circuits that have been reduced in Parkinson's disease. In a few people, this chemical jolt overrides the cortex and leads to full-scale hypersexual behavior."

"Sounds pretty technical for a little ole Dixie gal like me," said Mary Rose with a clear note of irritation basting her voice. "I'm happy. Why not just fix Sam's wonker?"

"I can't do it, Mary Rose. By protocol this type of side effect requires me to stop your new medicine."

In an instant Mary Rose's facial expression turned from hopefulness to despair. Her extensive protestations that followed proved futile. I had research criteria to abide by and could not be budged by her pleading. In addition, I worried that if left alone, Sam would become overtaxed and depressed and might physically collapse.

"How about for the next couple of weeks the two of you visit a counselor. You've had a major disruption in your lives caused by the experimental medicine. I'll see you back when Mary Rose has been off the new medicine for two weeks."

The clinic visit had concluded, but I worried for the next two weeks about Mary Rose and Sam and especially about the state of their relationship. I had grave doubts their bond would survive. Other than a sexual relationship and mutual loneliness, Mary Rose and Sam had little in common.

In the interim, I received rare reports from Cheryl. Mary Rose had called early on to verbally bludgeon her and to demand reconsideration of what she considered my "glaring mistake." She clearly missed her supercharged libido. Mary Rose had spoken to Cheryl graphically and uncharacteristically, I thought, for the southern girl she was. A smiling Cheryl later joked, "As good as Mary Rose makes it sound, maybe I need some of those pills."

The two weeks crept by with my anxiety amping up daily. Eventually Mary Rose returned for her appointment, accompanied, as requested, by Sam. On entering the exam room, I was heartened to see Sam wearing his soiled, rumpled Dallas Cowboys cap and dirty work boots. Mary Rose wore a short-sleeved linen sweater, tailored pants, diamond stud earrings, and a simple gold necklace. Her appearance contrasted with that of her prior visit. I interpreted their dress as a hopeful sign.

"Well, how's it gone?"

"Sure is different," Mary Rose said, scowling her displeasure at me.

"How's that?"

"You were right, about a day or two after stopping the new medicine, my libido crashed back to earth. Wow, that medicine was really good stuff. Can't say I don't miss it."

"Now, we are still messing around," Sam said, sounding

a little defensive. "Maybe once a week rather than imitating Spanish fly-munching prairie dogs."

"So how's the relationship going?" I asked.

"Since we ain't living in the bedroom all the time, found other things to do," Sam said.

"I hadn't known that Sam liked to bowl. I used to bowl in a league back in South Carolina. We've joined a league on Thursday nights."

"Also taken in some flicks and she drug me out to an opera. Still like my Country and Western music, least can understand what they're singing about." Sam grinned mischievously.

"Where are the two of you living most of the time?"

"Both in Lubbock and Muleshoe. Kind of getting used to Lubbock," Sam said. "Getting partial to these gourmet restaurants rather than having to eat my own cooking."

Mary Rose responded in kind. "I'm starting to like Muleshoe better than before. Now it is not high culture to be sure, but I've developed an interest in the history of Bailey County, the old Muleshoe Ranch, and the history of the railroads there. Have begun to care for the Mule Memorial that sits near the intersection of US 70 and 80. Did you know the town's name was taken from the old Muleshoe Ranch when the original rancher Henry Black found a mule shoe on his property? Always liked history; it must be in the blood of us southerners."

I noticed they sat next to each other and intermittently exchanged affectionate looks. Mary Rose patted Sam on the back of his gnarled hand. I took a deep sigh. I felt my concerns about Mary Rose and Sam's relationship evaporating. They had survived the calming of the drug-induced, libidinous storm, and their unlikely craft amazingly was still afloat.

I hesitated before leaving the exam room, turned, and inquired about their plans for the remainder of the day. Sam seemed anxious to share their agenda.

"Turns out, Mary Rose plays cards. Didn't know till bout ten days ago—too busy with other things, suppose. Had to teach her how to play pinochle."

Mary Rose said, "We play pinochle most days. Kind of our

own special afternoon routine. Sam really enjoys it, and I do too. And for some reason Sam always adjusts the table just so and makes big stacks of turkey and ham sandwiches, and pretty good ones at that, at least for an old cotton farmer."

I saw Sam Woodley drop his head and risk a furtive smile in my direction.

Chapter 11

# MIND SPARK

*Only in quiet waters things mirror themselves undistorted. Only in a quiet mind is adequate perception of the world.*

—Hans Margolius

"Gawd-awful weather," Dante drawled, momentarily interrupting his sweeping. His pile of rubbish lay in the corridor connecting the Health Sciences building to the University Medical Center Hospital.

"Good morning, Dante. Yes, almost as bad as Minnesota!" I always enjoyed my brief exchanges with Dante Rhodes since having treated him months earlier for his left foot drop. My gaze fell to his foot, where I noticed the absence of my prescribed foot-stabilizing prosthesis. Without it he was forced to step high in order to avoid tripping over his dangling foot. This unique characteristic gave Dante a recognizable gait and so distinctive that one wag referred to him as "that custodian, Hopalong Dante."

"Nothing but an old rusty barbed-wire fence 'tween here and the North Pole," Dante said, a gap-toothed smile enveloping his aged, milk chocolate–colored face. I heard Dante pronounce *barbed wire* as "bob warer" and nodded affirmatively.

Autumn gradually gives way to winter in most places, but not so on the Llano Estacado. There winter announces itself with shrieking "blue northers" and icy, bone-shuddering blasts of sleet and snow. Such a howler the previous day had stunned those of us living on the South Plains and had caused me to rummage through my closets in search of heavy coat, fur cap, woolen muffler, and fur-lined gloves. Minnesota had prepared me well for frigid weather.

Dante worked, nudging the pile of trash along with his broom. He hummed a slow, lyrical melody. My gaze settled on a red broken comb, several silver hairpins, and a flat rubber tourniquet among the dust pile. A thought nagged at me from deep within my brain. These objects looked strangely familiar. *Didn't I watch him sweeping up these very same objects recently?* Recognition of his guile struck me like a Taser. I could not avoid breaking out in a broad smile. I shook my head and winked knowingly, as I passed Dante by.

"Can't be running out of work, now kin I," said Dante, his honeyed words continuing to trail me down the echoing hall-way like a lonely puppy.

*Wish my letter of recommendation to the personnel department hadn't been quite so glowing. But with his neuropathy and his age, he needed a job, and no one else would have hired him.* This thought assuaged my somewhat guilty conscience.

Since moving back to Texas about a year earlier, I had gained experience and confidence in performing my work as an associate professor in the Department of Medical and Surgical Neurology. The large number of patients in need of neurological care and my heavy teaching responsibilities still burdened me, but overall I had found my job not only challenging but also enjoyable.

The clinical and teaching workload had worryingly caused me to neglect my research interests, creating pitfalls for my ultimate promotion and tenure. Several well-respected clinicians had failed to have their employment contracts renewed, despite having had glowing reviews of their teaching and patient-care activities. They had been forced to leave the medical school faculty due to insufficient numbers of scholarly articles. Publish or perish really does exist in academia.

The new medical school at Texas Tech lacked endowments and relied heavily on income from the physicians' practice plan. Perhaps no better option existed than to sacrifice good clinicians for the long-term benefit of the school, yet this forfeiture of human talent discomforted me. The threat of a similar fate gnawed at me like a hungry hyena.

Without employment, how would I support Trudy and my kids? How could I afford the large quantity of dog food required for Dice? How would we pay our mortgage at its sky-high rate of 19 percent?

But when confronted by the choice of a needy patient or hiding out in the research laboratory, I always chose to care for the patient.

*With the additional faculty we've been promised, I'll eventually be able to spend time on research. Plus, my newly hired nurse practitioner, Vicki, should free up more time for my research.*

Vicki Masters was an early adopter of the new system of medicine. In the 1980s, a few nursing programs had begun to turn out nurse practitioners willing to venture away from treating patients with sore throats and colds to instead assist specialists. I would lean on Vicki heavily over the next dozen years.

On hospital rounds that morning I documented my findings, wrote orders, and answered patients' questions. Two hours into rounds, my pager went off and directed me to call the emergency room. The physician in the ER described a confused and babbling man who had been brought from a nearby store on University Avenue. Doctor Mayfield requested I evaluate the young man, Robbie Marshall.

"Vicki, how about you check on this ER patient? I'll finish here and catch up—take me about half an hour." Vicki Masters, my nurse practitioner of several months, had moments before looked bored, staring out the window at the inclement gray weather. She had a mannerism of fiddling with her ever-present opinion buttons. That day her choice of button boasted, "My border collie is smarter than your honor student." Confronted by the waiting challenge in the emergency room, the diminutive Vicki sprang to life, her green eyes behind oversized rimless glasses twinkling with renewed enthusiasm.

"You got it, boss. Call as soon as I've scoped it out." She bustled down the hallway, sneakers squeaking and curly red hair bouncing at the nape of her neck. The pert Vicki was around five feet tall, weighed barely one hundred pounds, and exhibited nonstop freckles. She had a quick tongue, was hardworking, and knew the limits of her expertise. When expressing her views, she was about as subtle as a swarm of bees.

I appreciated Vicki for having joined me in my practice. The job was daunting and required long hours. It was not a job for the meek. But with her help, I had been getting home by seven o'clock rather than the previous nine o'clock or later. I also believed that together we provided better service for our patients.

I was in the process of completing my last chart note when my pager beeped. The pager said to call the emergency room and displayed the code number 29. Vicki had chosen 29 as her identifying code, maintaining her stated age would never exceed that number.

Within a few minutes, I arrived in the emergency room and encountered a clearly agitated and red-faced Vicki. While always talkative, she now blithered with so many seemingly unrelated utterances that I had difficulty comprehending her meaning.

"Whoa, Vicki, slow down. I can't follow what you're saying."

She took a deep breath and began in a more deliberate fashion.

"What's the penalty for decking a cop," she fumed, her green eyes spitting malice.

"What's up? What cop?" I stammered. She began to rave anew, with still more disparate sentences, pontificating about police brutality, the inalienable rights of the arrested, and how a sub-eighty IQ must be a requirement to join the Lubbock police force.

"Vicki, what's happening with the patient?" Exasperation basted my voice.

"Well, he's a twenty-six-year-old guy who just happens to be really, really cute. Got the lightest blue eyes, just like Paul Newman's, and this cute little cleft in his chin," she said, pointing to her tiny freckled chin for emphasis.

"Could you just tell me his symptoms?"

"Well, boss, he's in a PhD engineering program at Tech and got confused in a bookstore. His speech was not making sense to the manager. The manager became worried and wondered if he was on drugs or something, and called both the police and an ambulance. Kind of covered all his bases. Fortunately for my cute little engineer here, the ambulance arrived first."

Vicki had a habit of spritzing her words—a rapid verbal mannerism as unusual in slow-talking West Texas as palm trees. I always had to maintain close attention when she spoke and had long since forsaken trying to interrupt her. What's more, when she became involved in providing a medical history or telling a story, she had a way of losing track of what else was going on around her, once even mindlessly following me into the men's restroom. She had clearly, by this time, focused in on the case.

"I found this kid handcuffed by this beetle-browed Neanderthal with a badge who just happens to be packing a small cannon."

"Why handcuff a confused man who's speaking funny?" I asked.

"Beats me. Maybe the cop just got a new set and the missus didn't cotton to his idea of fun bedroom games!"

I glanced across the way into room 4, where I spotted a young man in his twenties lying on an exam table. His hands were cuffed in front of him. Beside him a dark-haired, burly, middle-aged police officer impatiently stood.

*Surely looking confused in a shop isn't illegal? Must be more to the story than that.*

Moments later, on entering the room, I introduced myself to the patient and the police officer. I set my black bag on the bedside table. The patient greeted me politely; the police officer grunted disdainfully.

"I'm Robbie Marshall," said the cleft-chinned, blond-haired

young man lying on the table. He shared he was from Houston and that he had almost completed advanced work in mechanical engineering. Robbie did not strike me as confused in the least. His height was hard to determine, but he possessed a slight build and had a pleasant, sincere way of speaking. I noted his plastic pocket protector with four different colored pens and several markers.

"How come you're wearing handcuffs?" I asked.

"Don't know, sir. Just blacked out, and when I came to, was in an ambulance with the big fellow here with the badge and wearing these." He gestured by slightly raising both hands.

Robbie Marshal gave Vicki an endearing smile and shrugged his shoulders. Vicki blushed, smiled shyly, and flicked her crimson tresses.

"The little peckerhead punched me," interjected the officer. I noticed his name tag read Ray Armstrong. On closer inspection I also noted that he had a swollen, soon to be black eye. The officer with what looked like a single connected eyebrow took a menacing step toward Robbie, projecting intimidation. I noticed the heady, overpowering scent of his cheap aftershave.

"You better tell the truth now and be quick about it, Marshall. And while you're at it, tell him how you popped me when I wasn't even looking." Officer Armstrong's voice was deep, overly loud, and uncompromising. Robbie gazed back at him pacifically.

Vicki stepped forward. "Buster, you touch him and I'll kick you so hard in a place where you'll never again have to worry about birth control." The officer's irritated face turned toward Vicki. I raised my hand in a sign of compromise and scowled at Vicki until she retreated a few steps.

"Robbie, if I get the officer to take off the cuffs, you promise to behave yourself?"

"Yes, sir, would appreciate it. Hurts my wrists."

"Come on, Officer. Can't perform a neurological examination with him like this."

I glanced at Vicki and saw her still glaring at the giant policeman. She shifted her feet from side to side, looking like a featherweight boxer waiting for the bell to ring. The feisty Vicki struck a vivid contrast to the ponderous police officer. The cop was formidable, standing at least six foot four and weighing more than 275 pounds. His belly bulged over his broad belt like an overfilled ice-cream cone. I observed a menacing black nightstick and large revolver attached to his thick, black leather belt. Officer Armstrong's bulk contrasted with the slightly built, decorous young man whom he had in custody.

*Looks like overkill to me.*

"Don't think we need those cuffs now," I persisted.

"I'm arresting this punk and putting his scrawny ass in jail, that is, if I can get him out of this emergency room sometime this century."

Vicki again got in the swarthy cop's face. "What's your problem, Bozo, you miss your donut stop this morning?"

"Look, Little Orphan Annie, you stay out of it. He's going downtown."

I moved between them. "Come on, Officer Armstrong, I really need to examine Mr. Marshall. Please take off the cuffs. I'll take full responsibility."

Only after explaining that our arguing was delaying his discharge from the emergency room did Officer Armstrong relent and remove the handcuffs. He then stationed himself at the doorway like Horatio at the bridge. I noticed him fingering his nightstick with what I interpreted as a wishful look on his fleshy face. I proceeded to ask the patient a few more perfunctory questions.

"Doctor, I really can't remember anything after entering the bookstore."

Officer Armstrong, with his jaw muscles bulging, finally could refrain no longer and butted into the conversation, claiming Robbie was flat-out lying.

I then asked Robbie to sit up on the side of the exam table. He readily complied. I began by checking for increased intracranial pressure by peering in his eyes with an ophthalmoscope. I went on to check his other cranial nerves, all of which were normal. I did a mental status examination: Robbie was alert, was cognitively intact, and complied promptly and courteously when questions were asked of him. He appeared genuinely perplexed by his absence of memory during the time he had spent in the bookstore. His muscle strength proved normal, as was his sensory examination.

All had gone well until about ten minutes into the examination. I opened my black medical bag and removed a reflex hammer. A light tap of the hammer showed his reflexes were normal. Then Robbie Marshall surprised me. "Why'd you hit me with that little hammer?" he asked. Checking reflexes was a routine part of a neurological examination, and the small rubber-tipped hammer that I had taken from my black bag would have caused him no particular discomfort. I gave a quick apology and shrugged it off. However, I noted a surprising amount of irritation rising in Robbie's voice.

A little later I was checking for a Babinski sign by lightly stroking the sole of his foot. "Hey, that hurts, Doc. Don't be scratching my foot again!" he demanded belligerently.

"Sorry, Mr. Marshall, just checking an important reflex. Would you mind too much if I checked the other foot?"

"Well, if you have to—but be quick about it," he snapped. I felt puzzled as to why his previous cooperative attitude had receded as quickly as had our fall weather the day before.

A few minutes later I began to examine his coordination. "Would you please touch your nose and then my finger?"

"Sounds like a stupid thing to do." His words were pressed and edgier. "Why don't you just bug out and leave me alone with this fat goon here?" Robbie's gaze now peered malevolently at Officer Armstrong.

"Oh, come on, Mr. Marshall, we're just about finished now," I cajoled.

Over a few short minutes, I had witnessed a definite change in Robbie's behavior. The progression had become worrisome. The initial polite, deferential, diffident attitude had evolved into an irritated, argumentative, openly truculent, and finally overtly hostile tirade.

"Trust me, we're finished." Robbie spat out his words angrily, balling his fists. I recoiled.

Robbie Marshall had by then evolved into a thoroughly troubling state. Nothing I had said or done seemed to explain his malice. Robbie's face then flushed, and he began to sweat profusely. I had difficulty understanding what I was observing and could not remove my gaze from his dramatically changing facial expression. Robbie's pupils dilated. His muscles tensed and his gaze narrowed to a hard, cold, and distant stare. His breathing mimicked Darth Vader's. His eyes filled with hatred.

I observed Vicki's eyes also widen, and she stopped moving distractedly, staring at Robbie with an astonished expression on her cherubic face. She began to twist a tight curl of red hair repeatedly around her finger. A smug look came over Officer Armstrong's his face as he slowly pulled the nightstick free from his belt. He gave a hearty laugh, his belly surging wavelike over his broad leather belt. I saw his knuckles whiten around the nightstick, as he struck the palm of his hand with little audible smacks.

"Ain't he just the little charmer, Doc? Now this is the Robbie boy I know and love."

"Now don't you be cracking this kid's skull. Doesn't need a head injury too," I said firmly.

"You stupid pigs, gonna kick your asses!" Robbie screamed.

I whipped my head around to see Robbie in a purple-faced fury, a primitive wrath of a sort that I never before witnessed. He expressed a primal fury that seemed to search the immediate environment for a ready target. I heard the approaching footsteps and excited voices of emergency room personnel. *Thank goodness the cavalry is coming.*

Robbie readied his body like a tiger preparing to spring. He gripped the table with both hands and bent forward at the waist, the metamorphosis completed from a quiet young man to a fearful, menacing beast. Suddenly the room felt far too small. Robbie sneered, and I heard him grind his teeth. He began to swing his fists and kick at me, causing me to stumble awkwardly backward.

"You bastards, you lousy bastards!" His words sounded slurred and almost inhuman. His escalation of anger proved frightful to watch, increasing like the buildup of a nuclear reaction.

Just then a loud, primal howl rose from deep within him. The unholy, ear-splitting cry did not sound as if it came from a man but from some primordial beast. Robbie's eyes stared straight ahead, his body stiffened, and he leaned precariously near the edge of the exam table.

I lunged toward him, wedging my body against the table, attempting to prevent him from pitching off the table. I even then was careful to stay clear of his grip. Blood-tinged foam from his mouth sprayed my face and clothing. Robbie arched his back mightily. His muscles contracted, and his body became board stiff. Seconds later large jerks of his arms and body began to occur. With effort I was able to drive into Robbie and push him back into the middle of the bed.

At last the origin of his dramatic change in behavior came clear. His convulsion lasted no longer than a minute but seemed an eternity. I struggled to hold him on the table. Vicki had crept up to assist me in preventing Robbie from falling. Curiously, in the meantime, the police officer had retreated from the room and had disappeared into the surging crowd of emergency room personnel that had gathered just outside the door.

Robbie's clothing was drenched with sweat. Finally his stiffening and jerking subsided and he fell limp, unconscious and spent. The only movement, other than the heaving of his chest, consisted of occasional droplets of bloody saliva escaping from the corners of his mouth. His breathing sounded harsh.

"Jeeesus, what was that?" bellowed Officer Armstrong, peering in through the doorway.

"Well, whaddaya know?" I said. "We saw something rare—a seizure beginning as an angry outburst, then developing into a full-blown rage attack before finishing as a generalized convulsion."

"Acted just like my ex, when I caught him boffing the babysitter," Vicki added in a private side comment to me.

"You're not telling me his fighting and cussing was him having a seizure?" asked the policeman, a puzzled look on his broad face.

"Well, the buildup of his anger was part of his seizure. Sometimes the seizure stops before building to a full convulsion. Just depends."

A look of partial recognition appeared on Officer Armstrong's perplexed face. After a few seconds he asked, "What's a seizure anyway?"

Since I needed to stay with Robbie during his postictal period, I went ahead and launched into an explanation. "It begins with an abnormal firing of brain cells, kind of like an electrical spark that kindles a fire that may or may not progress to a wildfire. Which brain cells fire off first determines the symptoms, such as funny sensations, abnormal movements, or even psychical experiences like we saw today. Robbie's seizure began in his limbic system, the emotional part of the brain, and caused him to suffer fear and rage. The spark spread throughout the brain, like a large fire building from a small one. The brain can sometimes inhibit the seizure spread, but it's not always successful at impeding its progression."

Officer Armstrong looked puzzled. "Well, I'll be damned, being a cop's getting more complicated every day." His attitude had altered and he appeared curious to learn more about Robbie's medical situation.

By the time Robbie Marshall regained full consciousness thirty minutes later, he had received an intravenous loading dose of phenytoin, an anticonvulsant. Within an hour the lagging, postseizure confusion had cleared, revealing his usual mild-mannered, respectful self.

After observing Robbie's seizure and recovery, Officer Armstrong began to harbor doubts about arresting him.

"That squeamish district attorney likely won't bring a case. Has a real soft spot for Tech students." Officer Armstrong still smarted from his black eye, and for it I could tell he still wanted to exact some price from Robbie. But as more time passed, like Robbie's confusion, the officer's resentment gradually subsided.

Vicki convinced Robbie to apologize to the police officer, even though Robbie claimed no recall of having ever struck the officer or having done anything wrong. I left the room for a few minutes to take a telephone call and on my return noticed Officer Armstrong and Robbie conversing about the inclement weather and the just completed Tech football season. They became animated in their storytelling and acted as if they were old chums. Officer Armstrong even shook Robbie's hand when he was preparing to depart.

"No hard feelings, Robbie? Well, good luck to you. Hope you find a good job. Make a bunch of money."

Later follow-up in the neurology clinic revealed Robbie's easygoing nature had never again fallen prey to seizures, so long as he regularly took his seizure medicine. No specific cause for his seizures was determined, and he was given a diagnosis of an idiopathic seizure disorder.

I have reflected on this incident, recalling how such events at times have a funny way of working out. That cop wasn't the brute Vicki and I initially suspected. At the outset we had clearly misjudged him. Robbie Marshall's spectacular change in behavior had at first stupefied Vicki and me, just as it had the officer. Only by witnessing the entirety of his seizure was I able to understand Robbie's violent behavior as being beyond his control, a fact that also had not been lost on Officer Armstrong. Also after witnessing Robbie's transformation, I better understood the police officer's anger and suspicions. During the time spent in the exam room, all our attitudes changed about as dramatically as the fifty-degree temperature drop the day before.

My understanding of people has increased by having practiced as a neurologist. The process of neurological diagnosis draws upon syndrome analysis. This diagnostic discipline has the doctor beginning with a single complaint and layering on additional clues. This allows for a steadily improving accuracy of diagnosis. In my experience, the initial clues frequently prove wrong or too incomplete to confirm a diagnosis. Only after additional medical history, neurological examination, and various diagnostic tests may the correct diagnosis become achievable.

In the same fashion, additional time and experiences often allow for better understanding of people. Being an impatient person, I strive to learn underlying motivational factors as people function within their own distinct physical and psychological environments. If I am able to do this, the outcome is almost always rewarding.

"Come on, Ray," said Vicki. "I'll buy you a mug of coffee and a couple of big old jelly donuts. That's one thing the cafeteria can cook without completely screwing it up. You look a might shaken, big guy, and it'll make you feel better. Besides I want to register a complaint about the city hassling my dog Fritz when he's off his leash."

As Vicki herded the police officer in the direction of the hospital cafeteria, she reminded me of a tug moving a blue-and-gold ocean liner. Ray's objections to Vicki's plan proved as fruitless as trying to whistle down the spring winds. As they departed, I heard the following exchange:

"But, miss, I don't know nothin' 'bout animal control."

"Ridiculous, Ray. You just hush now, and I'll tell you everything you need to know about animal control and the inherent worth and spirituality of animals, and I'll share what you should be doing as you cruise around our fair city to help out our furry friends."

*Chapter 12*

# CHOSEN ONES

*There is an elasticity in the human mind, capable of bearing much, but which will not show itself, until a certain weight of affliction be put upon it; its powers may be compared to those vehicles whose springs are so contrived that they get on smoothly enough when loaded, but jolt confoundedly when they have nothing to bear.*

—Charles Caleb Colton

**Help Wanted**
*Immediate opening to feed, bathe, dress, and manage a stubborn person with aggressive outbursts, middle-of-night terrors, and incontinence. Hours 24/7, 365 days/year without pay or benefits. No personal time off or sick leave. Offers heartbreak. PLEASE apply soon.*

Who would respond to such an advertisement? Yet as implausible as it sounds, family caregivers of Alzheimer's disease victims serve in precisely this capacity. These caregivers are the unsung heroes of medicine and deserve praise. The following story is my tribute to these essential and wonderful people.

"Mac's getting lost driving, have to tell him where to turn," said Judy Campbell. "Losing his memory for years, but needs help dressing. Soils himself, can't any longer pay the bills, and, well, most everything he does, needs a little dab of help from me."

Judy sat in my office, squirming in her chair. Gray roots peeked from beneath her curly, blond hair. Judy picked at her rose-colored fingernails while relating Mac's problems. At earlier visits she had told me these very same incidents. So while unenlightened by the complaints, I was surprised by her display of uncharacteristic nervousness.

In my opinion Judy was the poster child for homemaker, wife, and mother. Four decades earlier, following World War II, she had left an administrative position with the American Embassy in London to marry Mac Campbell, a kilted, mustachioed officer in the Highland Guard. To be sure, not all wartime marriages had been as successful, but this marital interweaving of Texas sagebrush and Scottish thistle had proven as strong as a heavy anchor rope. Since the Campbells' visit four months previous, Judy had lost weight and appeared more fatigued. Her face was gaunt and strained, and although her interaction with me was as warm as a toasted bun, she exuded less animation.

"It's not just that Mac's needs are so great, it's that someone has to be around all the time and supervise his actions," Judy said. "It's the constancy of the caregiving that wears me down."

Caregivers of persons suffering from Alzheimer's disease confront unexpected outbursts, troubling crises, and middle-of-the-night terrors, relying on their own instincts and diminishing reserves of energy. Nowhere in marriage contracts are these potential rigors spelled out. If they were, I fear marriage rates would plummet like a boulder rolling off a cliff.

Not only are the physical requirements strenuous, but also the diminished personhood of the afflicted makes the task even harder to sustain. Despite half a century of marriage, the spouse may one day peer across the breakfast table at her confused mate and hear the soul-crushing question, "Who are you?"

At the outset, the intricacies of caregiving are like the layering of the triple canopy of a rain forest, impossible at first to view in its entirety. Caregiver, family, and friends usually at the outset mercifully misunderstand the growing complexity of the caregiver's job.

In an all too random fashion, caregiving is thrust upon family members regardless of financial situation, psychological predispositions, or health status. Family caregivers, most often a spouse or child, usually end up punching above their weight class and soar above their own estimates of caregiving abilities.

"What's really bothering you today, Judy? You just don't seem yourself."

Judy Campbell dropped her head and sat motionless for a few seconds before responding. She took a deep breath. "Doctor Hutton, I should share something with you."

Her penetrating blue eyes studied me intently, searching my face for a sympathetic signal. Her fidgeting ceased. In her soft drawl Judy said, "The breast cancer from two years ago—well, it came back. My oncologist said it's already spread to my liver and bone marrow. I may have only months to live." Her voice had dropped to a barely audible whisper. After a brief pause, she continued. "I'm not overly concerned about myself, but I'm terribly worried about Mac. He can't make it without me." The plaintive, heartbreaking tone of this final statement struck me like a cresting tidal wave.

"Judy, I am so very sorry." I sat for a few moments, a sense of loss enveloping me. Judy Campbell impressed me as a special person who possessed an ever-present joy and zest for life. She had always seemed to draw on some vast, hidden reserve of courage. When faced with death, the emotional fortitude of the Judy Campbells of the world has always amazed me. How do some people benefit from an extra dollop of bravery to face life-altering events, while others collapse at the first tinge of a toothache?

"I suppose I've been helping Mac more than I'd realized," Judy said. "I worry what will become of him, after I'm gone."

Judy sat back in the powder blue winged-back chair in my office and lightly dabbed at her moist eyes with a tissue. Her glistening blue eyes had a pleading, vulnerable quality about them. While usually nicely dressed and coiffed, Judy's true beauty sprang from deep within her.

"We'll do everything possible to help you and Mac. Let's talk about this more."

We spent some time discussing her situation. I offered what Vicki, my nurse practitioner, liked to refer to as "sympathetic noises," although my commiserations were truly heartfelt. Eventually we returned to the subject of caring for Mac. I asked, "Judy, do you have any family or close friends who can help out with Mac?"

"Unfortunately," Judy replied, "our closest friends have either died or moved away to be nearer their families. Our only child, a son, lives on a small farm in Arkansas." She made a pained facial expression.

"Is there a problem with your son?"

"Well, we're not getting along; had a falling out when he divorced. Freddie became so bitter after his injury, ended up divorcing a wonderful girl and he was just so, so into himself. In fairness to Freddie, he suffered a near-fatal car crash that left him with difficulty walking and getting around. He now lives on his disability pension. But in a pinch, I think Freddie would help out his dad."

"Have you talked with Freddie recently and shared your sad news?"

Judy dropped her eyes. "I don't think Freddie understands how his dad has changed. I just haven't been able to bring myself to tell him. Freddie doesn't know about my cancer recurring either." A look of embarrassment crossed her face.

How often had I seen this scene play out? The spouse has failed to share her mate's deterioration or her near collapse with family members and then suddenly hits the wall, requiring urgent help. Often the collapse follows a florid middle-of-the-night incident.

I recall an eighty-year-old lady who slumped exhausted into my clinic one day after a night of cross-examination by her demented, paranoid lawyer of a husband. He had grilled her with full legal decorum during the wee hours the night before, as she had sat in a kitchen chair in her nightgown and furry slippers. Her husband had attempted to elicit a confession from her that their four sixty-something-year-old children had, in fact, all been illegitimate! Such challenges for caregivers become humorous only many years later and only with the benefit of substantial hindsight.

The person with Alzheimer's disease usually can hold it together when company arrives. It is later, during the long, disorienting nights, that crises commonly occur. While visitors notice memory loss and the retelling of old stories, they often miss the need for help with dressing and grooming, dealing with incontinence, and the stultifying paucity of original thought and novel conversation.

The loyal spouse, who often interjects answers to questions intended for the person with Alzheimer's disease, may even be viewed as overbearing. In actuality, this provides valuable face-saving for the Alzheimer's disease patient from his inability to answer the question. Or the Alzheimer's disease patient may refer questions to the spouse in a deft move to cover his memory loss. How frequently I have heard when asking someone with Alzheimer's a question, something like, "Well, I'll let the wife answer that one." For no matter how impaired, the potential for embarrassment for the Alzheimer's sufferer continues.

"Will you promise to contact your son, Freddie, and share your information about you and Mac?"

"I'll call Freddie, first chance I have," Judy said. She spoke with a note of resignation in her voice that caused me to believe she would follow through.

"I also want you to meet with Vicki, my nurse practitioner. She's really good about finding help for people."

I knew Vicki would identify social services and whatever other support might exist on the North American continent for Judy and Mac. She was just that way. Vicki would leave no resource untapped, as she never addressed any worthy task half-heartedly.

I must admit to also having harbored an ulterior motive. Vicki had recently returned from a "Save the Seals" rally in San Diego. Since returning, she had worn an oversized button picturing an angelic white baby seal. Helping Judy find resources, I thought, might distract Vicki from her nonstop efforts to stir up impressionable university students and papering the expansive Texas Tech campus with graphic "Outlaw Seal Hunting" posters. Vicki had a heart as big as Texas and a list of causes nearly as long as the state is wide.

A year or more passed without further contact with the Campbell family. One day Mac Campbell and a younger man entered my office. On meeting them in the exam room, Mac showed the joviality of the well-met traveling salesman that he had once been. He was wearing his tam-o'-shanter, having sported it since departing Scotland so many years earlier.

"Top of the day to ya," Mac said affably.

"It is good to see you, Mac. Is this your son?" I asked.

"'Tis indeed, and it's good to see ya, mon."

Mac offered his automatic snippet of speech in his lively, ear-caressing brogue. Freddie Campbell and I shook hands.

On mental status testing that day, Mac's dementia showed evidence of further progression. I gathered from the nurse's notes that his family physician was treating Mac with tablets to control hypertension. I confirmed Mac's high blood pressure and made a mental note to include his blood pressure values in my consulting letter to his family physician.

Mac Campbell's angular frame perched awkwardly in the small chair in the exam room, his elbows and knees protruding like sticks from a hastily built stork's nest.

"I notice your mom is not with you today," I said tentatively, fearing the worst.

"Afraid the cancer took her about six months back," said Freddie.

"I'm so sorry to hear that. She was an amazing and good woman."

Freddie said, "Her death was merciful at least. She died at home without much pain under the care of hospice in Abilene."

From this I derived a small degree of comfort. I would miss her graceful goodness. I saw Freddie's eyes well up with tears. I recalled the alienation that had existed between Freddie and his mother and noted Freddie's obvious warm feelings for her. I sensed reconciliation must have occurred.

Mac, to the contrary, appeared unfazed at the mention of his deceased wife of more than forty years. I knew Mac's lack of concern resulted from his deteriorated mental state and not from lack of love for Judy.

"Freddie, how have things gone with your dad?" I finally asked.

Freddie, dressed in blue jeans and a work shirt, leaned a cane over his thigh and sat thoughtfully for a few moments. This gave me time to notice that Freddie had inherited his mother's penetrating blue eyes. He had a slender build and infectious humor like his father.

"The situation's better than it was, but it couldn't have gotten much worse, I guess, unless the IRS had decided to audit me and the well had gone dry," Freddie replied, giving a game smile.

"How's that?" I asked.

Freddie shifted his cane and began to speak. "When Dad first came to live with me after Mom went into hospice, I figured he needed a warm place to live, a bit of food, and a little supervision. My jaw nearly fell out of its socket when Dad appeared one morning wearing his tam-o'-shanter, dress shirt, and necktie with his shirt tucked into his spotted, shorty-cotton pajamas. 'Dad,' I said, 'starting a new fashion trend this morning, are we?'

"I noticed that Dad had forgotten to shave portions of his face and was looking scruffy. It dawned on me that Mom must have been spending more time than I suspected sprucing him up." Freddie said he had still been mulling these surprises when his father took the pitcher of orange juice and poured it over his muesli. "Whoa, I thought," said Freddie, "my old Highlander's having a wee bit more problems than I suspected."

"What were you thinking at that point?" I asked.

"I realized then Mom's help wasn't just in the realm of advice. You know women—always like to tell a man how to run his life. I had rather suspected that was the case with Mom and Dad."

While Freddie Campbell had presented the events in a lighthearted fashion, I suspected learning his father's needs and caring for him had jarred him to the very depths of his emotional foundation.

"About a week later, I looked about the house and couldn't find the old Scotsman. I cruised about the farm in my Ford pickup and found him traipsing through the south pasture. Didn't appear upset or nothing, but pretty clear he didn't know his way back to the house."

"Could you tell what he was doing?" I asked.

"Said he was making sales calls. Imagine that? Had him a handful of paper, called 'em his order forms, pretty confused he was.

"Try as I might, I'm unable to keep Dad in the house. He's a crafty and resourceful old fellow—picks locks and crawls through windows."

On questioning I learned that Freddie's physical limitations had prevented him from accompanying his dad on walks. "Will your dad do what you ask?"

"Would if he could remember what I'd asked. Always gone along with the flow. Never loses his positive view of life, a real affable guy and always wants to please."

"That's a great sign, Freddie. The best predictor of how someone's personality will evolve with his illness is how he has dealt with earlier reversals in life. Sounds like your dad should cope well with his Alzheimer's disease."

"That's hopeful. I'd worried that he might become belligerent like some."

"So what if your dad escapes from the house?" I asked.

"We've had a mongrel dog adopt us. Just showed up at the farm. I've taken to sending the dog along with Dad. The dog knows his way back and, in a pinch, I think the dog could lead Dad to the house."

My attention then shifted to Mac Campbell, who stared vacantly at the wall. I asked Mac what he recalled of the events Freddie had described. It was evident Mac had not followed the conversation and had no recall of the occasion in question. "Well, Mac, what have you been up to lately?" I asked.

"I make me sales calls, and Buddy and I get in a spot of ball playing," said Mac ebulliently.

"Who's Buddy?"

"Buddy is the brown mongrel that accompanies Dad. The two have become as close as peanut butter and jelly," Freddie said.

Mac's eyes sparkled with obvious interest when Freddie spoke of Buddy.

"Sounds like a smart dog," I said.

"Smart and loyal. Each day they play fetch or a made-up version of baseball," said Freddie. "They wander around the farm and get a little exercise, enjoy themselves, I think. At night Buddy curls up at the foot of Mac's bed. They're inseparable."

"How are you taking to being a caregiver?" I asked.

"Must admit, feeling inadequate at times. Never thought I'd be picking out my Dad's clothes, shaving him, or wiping his bottom."

"How's his bowel and bladder control?" I asked.

"A few accidents, now and again," Freddie said with an embarrassed look crossing his face.

"Yes, I'm sure having to clean him up must make you feel odd. But he must have done the same for you years back?"

"I remind myself of that now and again. But this caregiving stuff makes me feel like an elephant trying to learn how to roller skate."

His comment prompted a discussion of strategies for dealing with Mac's more bothersome problems and the potential of still more challenges ahead.

I was surprised when a smile came across Freddie's face.

"Doctor, I had one idea that worked out pretty good."

"Tell me, Freddie."

Freddie gathered himself and began to tell his story. "Dad has always loved the American game of baseball. My Arkansas farm is too far removed to receive the Saint Louis Cardinals radio broadcast. They are Mac's favorite team. So I obtained an audiotape of a particularly exciting ball game. Each night after dinner, I load it into the tape player and turn it on for Dad. Every replaying of the game for Mac is a novel experience."

"What a great idea. His memory loss actually is a positive here for his enjoyment," I said.

"I even know just where he's at in the game without being in the room. In the bottom of the sixth inning, the Cardinals hit a home run, causing Dad to let out a hearty war whoop or applaud loudly. You'd think William Wallace was alive and well in the hills of Arkansas! In the top of the eighth, the opposing team beats out an infield ground ball for a base hit. A bench-clearing rhubarb breaks out. The radio announcer describes the Cardinals' coach and the first-base umpire as standing nose-to-nose, jawing animatedly at each other. Dad never fails to jump out of his chair and unleash a tirade of Scottish profanity. Even Buddy gets excited and begins to run around the room and bark."

"Freddie, that's a clever idea," I said. Freddie beamed, his self-assurance having been restored.

"When the game is over, Mac and Buddy head off down the hallway. Dad goes to bed contented that his Cardinals have won another close one."

"What a wonderful way to send your father off to bed," I said.

"Must admit listening to the same game over and over gets a little old. It's driving me a bit crazy actually. Suspect by now even the dog could call the play-by-play."

I chuckled, visualizing a dog sitting behind a bank of microphones. Insightfully, Freddie had recognized Mac's poor memory and had turned his memory loss into an opportunity for recurring enjoyment.

Many months passed of clinic encounters and daily patient problems that crowded out all thoughts of the Campbell family. Then one day I received a manila envelope with a neat hand-written return address from a small town in Arkansas. The letter was from Freddie and represented for me a welcome communication, notifying me of Mac's status. Each patient is like a book. To miss the last episodes of a patient sequel is like failing to read the final chapters of a suspense thriller.

With anxious hands, I tore open the letter and began to read. Freddie wrote in his surprisingly readable hand:

*Dear Doctor Hutton, Vicki, Cheryl and Staff,*

*Since you have played such an important part in our lives these recent years, I wanted to share a bit of information about Mac's final days. My mother and I appreciated the care Mac received at the Alzheimer Institute.*

*About a month ago, I rose early to fix our breakfast. When it was ready, I was surprised that my dad had not gotten up, being the early riser he is. Finally I went into his bedroom and, to my surprise, found his bed undisturbed. I searched the house but could not locate Dad. Eventually I went to the back porch and peered down the hill. A chocolate-colored object in the distance caught my eye, as it stood out from the green background.*

*Having little choice, I grabbed my two canes and trekked off down the hill, once almost falling. At the bottom of the hill and on parting the foliage, I saw the brown object to be Buddy, our dog. The dog just stared at me with his sad eyes and then pointed his nose toward a shallow ravine that lay not far beneath him. When I walked over, I found, as if asleep, the body of my old Dad, his tam-o'-shanter nearby. Mac was lying peacefully on his back, lifeless eyes staring at the morning sky. His face had a serene expression. The brown dog whimpered softly and hovered protectively over Mac's body. I had a hard time dragging Buddy away from my dad.*

Despite Mac Campbell's misfortune at developing Alzheimer's disease, I felt him fortunate to have received loving care from both Judy and Freddie. Each had made Mac's final days as pleasant and independent as possible.

Freddie's letter continued:

> In Mac's last two years, he had another helper, a four-footed one named Buddy who had wandered onto the farm and adopted Mac. He became a target for Mac's always-generous affection. Buddy was Mac's constant companion and never failed to lead Mac home from their walks. Now looking back, I've come to think of Buddy as an angel dog. I think the dog came to live with us for the purpose of looking after my old Dad. I am ever so grateful for this gift.
>
> I wouldn't say this caregiving stuff was ever easy. Wouldn't wish it even on an Englishman. But I can say that I've learned something about myself. I found I could do some pretty unpleasant things, like parenting my own father, changing his diapers, trimming his bushy mustache, and looking out for him. I never imagined I could have done these things. Never thought I had it in me. I guess it is just like the old saying, "Life is a dance. If you're smart you learn the steps."
>
> Got me to thinking about how much my parents put into raising me and setting me on the right path. I guess it taught me what unconditional love is really all about. Made me realize I had gotten bitter about life, and when I compared my life to others, I really had it pretty good.
>
> We buried Mac last month at the base of the hill. That was a special place for him and a place where he and Buddy spent a lot of time, looking out over the stock pond. Buddy and I frequently visit his grave.
>
> Buddy and I have also begun volunteering at a local Alzheimer's daycare center. Buddy's become quite the hit. He makes his rounds every day, letting people pet him, talk to him, and give him treats. I find it amazing how old, lifeless eyes begin to sparkle when Buddy drops his droopy muz-

*zle in their laps. Figure we both have learned something about Alzheimer's disease, and what we have learned might just help others. I somehow now feel a need to share what I learned from my old Scotsman. It's like he left me with one final gift.*

*I am reassured that Dad died peacefully and with his ever-faithful dog, Buddy, nearby. Oh, and I wanted to let you know that the night before Mac died, he heard the Cardinals win another one.*

In a metaphor that I found strangely comforting and moving, Freddie concluded his letter:

*I believe his companion, Buddy, must have been the one to call the final inning of Mac's last trip around the bases, as my dad looked into the sky for the Cardinals' winning home run.*

*Sincerely,*
*Freddie Campbell*

I folded Freddie's letter slowly and placed it back in its envelope. I felt my eyes water and my vision blur. I sat and reflected for a few minutes, contemplating the changed lives of Freddie, Judy, and Mac Campbell. Alzheimer's disease had altered each of their lives in unexpected and unpleasant ways. But as a result both Judy and Freddie had developed into amazing caregivers. Freddie had plumbed the depths of his being to mine hidden strengths previously unknown to him. Judy had served Mac with selfless devotion as long as her physical strength had allowed. The dog, as if by divine intervention, had arrived at Freddie's farm to provide support and companionship for the old Scotsman. How often I had heard from other families about their dogs becoming focal points for their Alzheimer's family members and how the dogs had provided faithful service, security, and constant reassurance.

Along with the letter, Freddie also enclosed a poem by a former senator from Freddie's nearby state of Missouri:

*The one absolutely unselfish friend that man can have in this selfish world, the one that never deserts him, the one that never proves ungrateful or treacherous, is his dog. . . . He will kiss the hand that has no food to offer; he will lick the wounds and sores that come in encounter with the roughness of the world. . . . When all other friends desert, he remains.*

—George G. Vest

*Chapter 13*

# DID ADOLF HITLER'S PARKINSON'S DISEASE AFFECT THE OUTCOME OF WORLD WAR II?

*The brain is the ultimate organ of adaptation. It takes in information and orchestrates complex behavioral repertoires that allow human beings to act in sometimes marvelous, sometimes terrible ways.*

—Jack P. Shonkoff and Deborah A. Phillips

I worked as a physician for forty years. In addition to my clinical practice, once Vicki was on board, I finally found time to do the research that was also to be part of my career at the university. Later, when entering private practice, I hired Jerry Morris, who greatly expanded my efforts in research. Research was a fulfilling endeavor, and Parkinson's disease was the focus of much of my work. One of my more captivating investigations regarded the alleged Parkinson's disease of Adolf Hitler.

The public's long-standing fascination with Hitler became evident for me in 1999 when I presented two scientific papers at an international medical conference in Vancouver, British Columbia. My first paper, on eye movements and Parkinson's disease, was carefully crafted and painstakingly presented, representing twenty years of my research. While politely received, the paper, I fear, was soon forgotten.

My second, more speculative presentation, I had developed over the prior six months. It dealt with Hitler's Parkinson's disease and how his illness might have influenced the Battle of Normandy. My Hitler presentation, to my amazement, created great enthusiasm and immediately went viral. The next morning my conjectures appeared on the front pages of newspapers around the world, and I quickly landed on a major Canadian morning television show. I became inundated by emails and calls from journalists. Newspapers in Europe trumpeted my contention that Hitler's Parkinson's disease–related behavioral changes contributed to the defeat of the Axis forces at the Battle of Normandy.

A British film studio (Brighton Films) later contacted me and asked me to assist in producing a documentary on Hitler's medical problems (showing in the United States at the time of this writing on the History channel, entitled *High Hitler*).

More recently I participated in another TV documentary on a similar topic. This program appeared on the United Kingdom's channel 4 as *Hitler's Hidden Drug Habit* and in the United States on the National Geographic channel and is titled *Hitler the Junkie*. Never before or since has a scientific contention of mine so quickly entered the general consciousness. Such is my personal experience and surprise with the resilient impact of *der Führer*.

Adolf Hitler, of course, was never my patient nor did I personally know him. But the huge impact he had on the world and the significant effect I believe his Parkinson's disease had on his life makes this account too substantial and historically important not to include in this collection of stories.

I have seen thousands of patients with Parkinson's disease, including many with the cognitive changes of advanced Parkinson's disease and even some who had similar personality types to Adolf Hitler. I also have had numerous conversations with Parkinson's disease patients who shared their innermost feelings and frustrations with me. Their honest reactions allow me to speculate about what life must have been like for Hitler as he dealt with this progressive disease.

To outsiders, the claim that Hitler had Parkinson's disease may seem outlandish, unfounded, and preposterous. But please, withhold your judgment until the end. Parkinson's disease is commonly diagnosed with visual observation. I have observed thousands of people with Parkinson's disease and many others without its telltale characteristics. In my initial research I had seen Hitler display many of these signs. Then, from a neurological colleague, Abe Lieberman, I gained an expanded appreciation for the medico-historical work on Hitler. I began to watch old videos of Hitler with my practiced neurological eye. I watched Hitler's stooped and shuffling walk, observed his hand tremor, viewed his failing to swing his left arm when walking, noted his blank facial expression, and imagined how the Parkinson's disease–related muscle stiffness must have felt. I visually examined Hitler in the same fashion that I used on a daily basis in my clinic to examine my own patients, and concluded he did indeed suffer from Parkinson's disease. Many other experts in Parkinson's disease concur. Thus I feel qualified to make these observations about Hitler's life and how his Parkinson's disease may have impacted his consequential and fateful decision making.

Hitler's medical issues are no excuse for his cruelty, nor should they be considered alone in attempts to understand his abhorrent actions. The Nazi era must be considered in its full social and political context even to begin to understand the forces at work. Nevertheless, his Parkinson's disease and other health issues also warrant full consideration. Hitler was, and still is, something of a historical enigma. Trying to understand the Nazi leader's mentality has today become the holy grail of World War II historians. Following my own research on Hitler, I have come to believe that too little attention has been focused on his health problems and their impact on his war-related actions.

For years Parkinson's disease research failed to address the behavioral aspects of this principally movement disorder. This behavioral area particularly interested me. Two of my colleagues in our large Parkinson's Center, Dr. Matt Lambert and Janet Schwantz, found characteristics of a mild frontal lobe syndrome that was uniformly present in patients who had had Parkinson's disease for ten years or longer. It is well accepted that frontal lobe dysfunction impairs the ability to plan, execute, and determine effectiveness of decisions. Our research results enticed me to review the Hitler literature and do the math for his disease duration. I wanted to learn whether or not Hitler was likely cognitively impaired by his Parkinson's disease at any stage during World War II.

To determine this, I first needed to establish the onset of Hitler's Parkinson's disease. Although I found various dates suggesting its onset, Lieberman made the most persuasive determination. Using Lieberman's postulated onset date of 1933, which he based on videotape evidence, by the Battle of Normandy in 1944 Hitler would have had Parkinson's disease beyond the meaningful ten years. *Aha!* Might Hitler's neurological illness explain his planning shortcomings (executive dysfunction) and clarify, at least in part, some of his ruinous strategic mistakes? This possibility prompted me to review the available evidence once more and led me to some surprising conclusions.

Join me now in meeting and getting to know this patient, Adolf Hitler, beginning with his birth and development and then his time in Vienna and the military. This chapter will provide evidence for his Parkinson's disease–related motor and behavioral alterations and the substantial impact his brain disorder may have had on his decision making. This "medicine of history" even raises the question as to whether Hitler's Parkinson's disease was sufficient to have altered the outcome of World War II.

### The Early Years
No one gazing into the angelic blue eyes of the infant born on the twentieth of April, 1889, in the northern Austrian border town

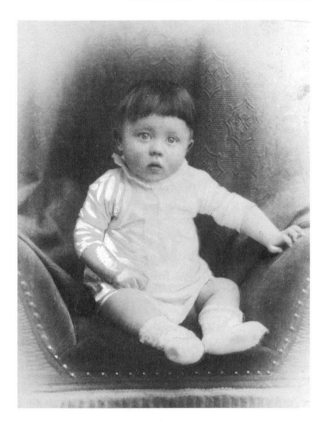

Adolf Hitler as a baby
(*Bundesarchiv*, Bild
183-1989-0322-506)

of Braunau am Inn could have fathomed the depravity that baby boy would one day release on the world. Adolf Hitler's birth was little noted at the time but would ultimately lead to the death of more than fifty million people. If an infant is a *tabula rasa*, then to interpret Hitler's life requires an understanding of his youth and development.

According to Fritz Redlich in his excellent psychiatric analysis *Diagnosis of a Destructive Prophet*, Alois Hitler, Adolf's father, was a fifty-two-year-old, alcoholic, doctrinaire customs officer at the time of Adolf's birth. His mother was twenty-nine-year-old Klara Hitler. Klara first worked as Alois's servant before serving as a nursemaid for Alois's tuberculous wife. She became Alois's mistress and ultimately married him and became his third wife.

According to Redlich, Adolf provided a revealing sentiment

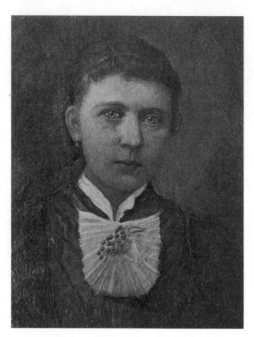 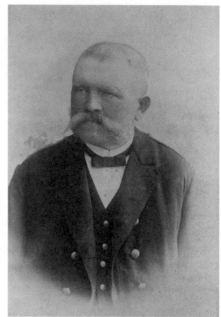

Klara and Alois Hitler, Adolf's parents (Library of Congress, LC-USZ62-74838, LC-USZ62-44196)

about his parents in *Mein Kampf*: "I honored my father, but I loved my mother." Young Adolf feared his father, an authoritarian, demanding, and at minimum, verbally abusive parent. Alois's scorn and humiliation of the sensitive boy undoubtedly damaged Adolf's personality development. Alois exhibited an uncompromising stubbornness that can later be easily discerned in his famous offspring. In contrast to his feelings for his father, Adolf adored his mother, who fawned affection on him. From Klara, Adolf gained a charming social demeanor that would later serve him well as a politician.

Adolf's full siblings, Otto, Gustav, Ida, and Edmund, all died young, causing Klara immeasurable grief. These tragic losses impelled her to dote even more on young Adolf. His troubled relationship with his undistinguished half brothers and sisters from his father's previous marriages proved ambivalent, if not downright hostile.

Young Adolf demonstrated acceptable performance in the country elementary school, but his middle school performance was poor. According to Franz Jetzineger, despite Adolf's high intelligence, he failed the first year of *Realschule* (secondary school) both in mathematics and natural history and earned low marks for conduct and diligence. He was forced to repeat the year. He again flunked mathematics in the second level of middle school and received low scores in conduct and diligence. Adolf then failed French in the third year but eventually passed a makeup examination.

One of Adolf's principal teachers, Eduard Huemer, commented on his prominent stubbornness. In addition to Adolf's talent for drawing, Huemer noted Hitler's inconsiderateness, self-righteousness, and tendency toward rage—all behavioral characteristics that would become more evident later in his life.

Hitler's reaction to the death of his mother may be revealing both for his development of anti-Semitism and his emotional dependence on her. In the winter of 1906–1907, Klara Hitler became very ill. Doctor Eduard Bloch, a Jewish general physician, diagnosed her with breast cancer. Klara underwent surgery at a local hospital, with Doctor Karl Urban as surgeon. Doctor Bloch continued to treat her for a postoperative chest infection by repeatedly packing it with iodoform gauze. During the fall of 1907 despite all medical efforts, Klara's health deteriorated and she died.

According to Rudolph Binion, a psychoanalytical historian, Hitler's anti-Semitism resulted from his opinion that Bloch had mistreated his mother by using too much iodoform gauze, by failing to provide pain relief, and by overcharging. However, Redlich drew a different conclusion. Based on Hitler's later grateful references to Doctor Bloch and his acknowledgment of his mother's poor prognosis from the outset, Redlich doubted Bloch played a major role in ramping up Hitler's anti-Semitism.

It was widely reported that Hitler had a Jewish ancestor. After an extensive search, Redlich concluded that no compelling evidence existed that Hitler's father was half Jewish, as some have speculated. But even after achieving ultimate political power in 1933, Hitler remained so troubled by this possibility that he obtained investigations by the SS (not too surprisingly reporting *der Fuhrer* had a completely Aryan background) and by his private attorney (the original report is no longer available, and the attorney's later musings on the subject are confusing). If in his own mind Hitler had been convinced of Jewish blood coursing through his veins, then his horrific anti-Semitic actions can be viewed as an overwrought defense mechanism (in psychoanalytical terms, reaction formation) toward his presumption of a shameful Jewish ancestry.

### Disappointment and Shame in Vienna and Military Service

After his expulsion from *Realschule* in 1904, Adolf moved to Vienna a year later. There he lived a bohemian existence, supporting himself with a state orphan's pension and financial help from his mother. Both in 1907 and 1908, Adolf applied for admission to the Academy of Fine Arts but received rejections in both instances. The academy's refusals cited "unfitness for painting" and advised Adolf to seek training in architecture. His lack of a diploma from the *Realschule* and his insufficient preparation prevented Adolf from even making an application to the architecture school. At that point his vocational aspirations hit a dishonorable and, I imagine, galling dead end.

In the midst of this humiliation, his beloved mother died from her breast cancer. This crushing loss exacerbated Adolf's melancholy and cut off his main source of affection. To make matters worse still, a court in Linz ordered him to turn over his orphan's benefits to his half sister, Paula. Even greater financial desperation then pursued Adolf. To survive, the nineteen-year-old began copying scenes from postcards and hawking them to tourists. At this financially and emotionally precarious stage of his life, Adolf was orphaned, penurious, and as adrift as a rudderless boat on the Danube.

Hitler claimed it was during this lonely and desperate period that he became an anti-Semite. In Vienna he first encountered a large Jewish community. Adolf developed fixed views that the Jews were enemies of Aryans and responsible for Austria's political and economic crises. By the conclusion of the Vienna period, Adolf had well-established personality characteristics of stubbornness, anti-Semitism, egoism, and cruelty. He later expressed his opinion that Jewish influence led to Germany's defeat in World War I. Hitler added to his anti-Semitism by blaming the Jews for playing principal roles in developing communism, a political philosophy he detested.

When World War I began to threaten, Hitler refused service in the Austrian army but jumped at the opportunity to join the German army. This apparent contradiction can be viewed as a psychological jab at his father, Alois Hitler, who was a proud Austrian and often berated his son to act in accordance. I can only imagine the personal satisfaction that Hitler must have felt years later in 1938 when Germany annexed Austria. At last he had one-upped his doctrinaire, abusive, Austria-loving father.

In the German army, Hitler rose to the rank of corporal and received decorations for bravery for running messages while under fire among German positions. In spite of suffering the trauma of war and personal injury in an English mustard-gas attack, Hitler for the first time experienced a sense of belonging to something larger than himself. During his hospital stay to recover from mustard-gas-induced blindness, he learned that Germany had sued for peace. Hitler was mortified by this news, creating in him a deep sense of rage that would fuel his political activism.

Following World War I and his recovery from the mustard-gas attack, Hitler moved to Munich. There he immersed himself in political issues with the nascent National Socialist Workers Party. His remarkable oratorical skills soon led to his meteoric rise within the party's leadership.

### The Onset of Hitler's Parkinson's Disease
Determining the onset of Hitler's Parkinson's disease proves important to my thesis. While dating the beginning of any chronic

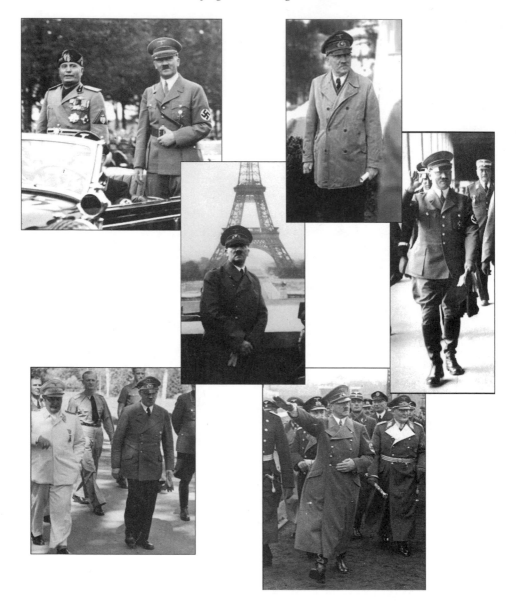

Adolf Hitler montage showing characteristic positioning of left hand and holding objects in his left hand, both approaches helpful for suppressing his tremor (*Bundesarchiv*, Bild 183-C13371, Bild 183-H12940, Bild 102-02192A, Bild 146II-728, Bild 183-2006-0810-500, Bild 146-1977-149-13; and US National Archives)

illness can be tricky, Parkinson's disease, more than others, readily reveals itself to visual observation.

Werner Maser, a German historian and journalist, described a transient tremor of Hitler's left hand as early as 1923 in association with the Beer Hall Putsch, Hitler's unsuccessful attempt to overthrow the Bavarian government that resulted in his prison stint for treason. Maser's claim followed his discovery of Hitler's medical records from 1905 to 1945. More convincing is Liebermann's contention based on 1933 films showing Hitler's failure to swing his left arm when walking, a common presentation for Parkinson's disease. Hitler was forty-four years old in 1933.

A 1934 snippet of film shows a tremor of his left hand during a Nuremberg rally. To an experienced eye, this clip, although brief, is compelling evidence for a Parkinson's tremor. In later years, this left hand tremor would become the most obvious visual sign of his disease.

A number of neurological authors, including me, have studied videos from later in Hitler's life and have found convincing evidence for Parkinson's disease. In my research I have found videos that show the classic Parkinson's disease manifestations: stooped posture, short-stepped gait, pill-rolling hand tremor, slow movement, micrographia, and the typical stony facial expression.

Hitler's positioning of his left hand is also subtly revealing. He adopted the mannerism of holding his left hand against his waist, or gripping his belt, or fingering objects with his left hand. Films show him holding his gloves or a rolled piece of paper. These are common and useful methods that people with Parkinson's disease employ as a trick to suppress hand tremor. I have witnessed this tactic many times with my own patients who described how this inhibits the embarrassing tremor.

### Impact of Hitler's Health on Operation Barbarossa
Historians and journalists continue to debate strategic questions relating to World War II. These questions have always captivated me. Had the Nazis somehow avoided making certain strate-

gic mistakes, would the ultimate outcome of the war have been different? Two important questions stand out for me: first, what caused Nazi Germany in 1941 to prematurely attack the Soviet Union, and second, what led to the delay of the German counterattack at the Battle of Normandy? Historians, debating these points, agree that the timing of Operation Barbarossa, the invasion of the Soviet Union by German military forces, would have been more successful if delayed from 1941 until 1944. Also, an earlier strong counterattack by German forces at Normandy on June 6 or 7 of 1944, especially at Omaha Beach, would have likely led to a different outcome of the battle. I believe these major strategic errors can be understood in light of Hitler's health concerns.

The ill-timed attack on the Soviet Union in 1941 occurred prior to Germany defeating the British, securing an alliance with Japan, replenishing its stockpile of conventional weapons, and developing to a war-ready status its rocket program, advanced submarines, jet airplanes, and other advanced and qualitatively superior instruments of warfare. Jet airplanes, remotely controlled rockets, and sound-tracking torpedoes were not planned for mass production until 1944.

Few would dispute the notion that Germany would have been stronger militarily a few years later than it was in June of 1941. Early in 1941 Hitler became obsessed with the view that he did not have long to live. I speculate that Hitler's health concerns and egomania played important roles in his decision to launch an early attack on the Soviet Union. I believe Hitler heard his own mortality ticking, ticking that was constantly reinforced by his Parkinson's-related movement and behavioral disorder. The German chancellor also suffered from advancing coronary artery disease that may have contributed to his sense of urgency.

Adolf Hitler would have had Parkinson's disease for eight years at the time of Operation Barbarossa. We can speculate on the severity of his illness by that date by reviewing the usual progression. Parkinson's disease advances fairly predictably,

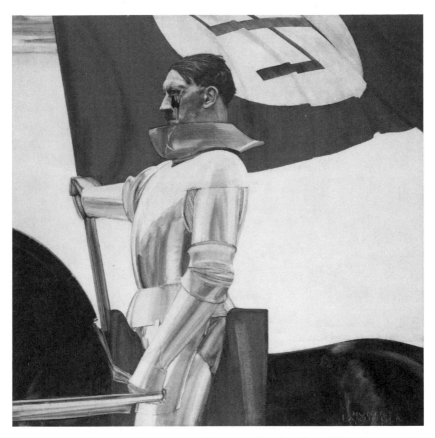

Nazi propaganda poster depicting Hitler as a gallant knight in full armor astride a black horse. In reality Hitler had never been on a horse. (Reprinted with permission of Erich Lessing/Art Resource, NY)

especially when untreated. It usually begins on one side of the body and, after a year or two, extends to the opposite side. The disease manifests with muscular rigidity, increased tremor, and progressive slowness of movement. By eight years a patient's independence, walking, and balance are typically reduced. In addition, the voice of a person with eight years of disease is usually soft and muffled.

Beginning in 1934, Hitler served as the supreme leader in Germany. The Nazi Party, through a massive propaganda campaign, encouraged the citizenry to view him in godlike terms.

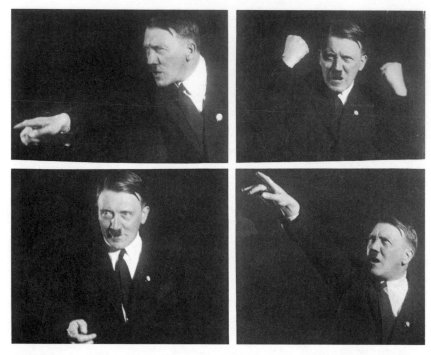

Adolf Hitler practicing gesticulations in front of a mirror (*Bundesarchiv*, Bild 102-10460)

Hitler was an egoist who wished to epitomize the Aryan race. Imagine the impact on his self-image when he began to spill food onto his clothing, encountered difficulty tying his own shoelaces, and experienced clumsiness when retrieving coins from his pocket. These are all frequent nuisances experienced by my own patients and likely proved especially disconcerting to Hitler. Perhaps even more vexing for Hitler would have been deterioration in his previously highly effective speaking voice.

At his peak during the early and mid-1930s, Adolf Hitler was said to have been the greatest orator of the twentieth century. He had a hypnotic verbal persuasiveness and well-practiced gesticulations that added immensely to his personal magnetism, connecting him to the German people.

Albert Speer was one of Hitler's closest colleagues. He spent much time with Hitler reviewing architectural plans for structures to be built following World War II and in his work as armaments minister. His observations prove especially helpful. In *Inside the Third Reich*, Speer's memoir, he described Hitler's voice toward the end of the war as becoming wavering and having lost its old masterfulness. Its force, he said, had given way to a faltering, toneless manner of speaking. What a blow to the Third Reich when Hitler's Parkinson's disease robbed him of his persuasive voice and broke his powerful bond with the German people.

Albert Speer further described Hitler's appearance toward the end of the war in unmistakably parkinsonian terms: "His limbs trembled; he walked stooped with dragging footsteps. . . . His uniform which in the past he had kept scrupulously neat, was often neglected in the last period of his life and stained by the food he had eaten with a shaking hand."

In the face of this deterioration, Hitler must have felt his mortality bearing down on him like a speeding Soviet heavy locomotive. During the final years of his life, his public appearances became severely constrained, and films and newsreels of him required careful censoring to expunge signs of his Parkinson's disease.

Keeping in mind that Parkinson's disease signs are an oft-employed visual and literary device to depict aging and frailty, what anathema for the supreme leader of the Third Reich to appear so depleted. What a shock it would have been if the German nation had realized that Hitler was no superman, but instead was a prematurely aging, frail, and tremulous mortal.

Due to his perception of failing health and diminishing vigor, Hitler had strong incentives to hasten the timetable for Operation Barbarossa. I speculate he recognized that his poor health limited the time he had to accomplish his conquests. By 1941 Hitler would have already lived the expected eight years, the average survival rate in the 1940s for a person with Parkinson's disease. His decision to invade early, once made, would prove to be an appalling strategic mistake.

## Morell's Belated Diagnosis and Treatment

Theodor Morell served as Hitler's personal physician and kept his own medical records. As a general doctor with special interest in venereal diseases, he knew little about neurological illnesses. Morell for years ignored or overlooked symptoms and signs of Parkinson's disease. Despite his relative lack of medical sophistication and his virtual shunning by Hitler's cadre of better-trained physicians, Morell nevertheless enjoyed Hitler's complete trust.

Morell deviated from the standard medical practice of the day, telling Hitler his importance to Germany required the inherent risks of using unproven, anecdotal therapies. I also believe Hitler was desperate and wished to try whatever looked to promise his continued leadership role.

Leonard and Renate Heston in *The Medical Casebook of Adolf Hitler* posit Morell provided amphetamines that eased Hitler's sense of fatigue, the most common symptom of Parkinson's disease. In the short term, amphetamines cause an outpouring of dopamine in the brain that elevates mood and improves the motor aspects of Parkinson's disease. Hitler would have welcomed and likely even demanded such a beneficial effect. Chronic use of amphetamines, however, increases the risk of a person developing Parkinson's disease and may have aggravated Hitler's neurological disorder.

The Hestons suggest Hitler may have developed a dependence on amphetamines, an eventuality that would have further secured Hitler's ongoing need for his controversial doctor. An additional consideration is that chronic amphetamine use frequently leads to great suspiciousness and paranoia. Such an abnormal mind-set would not have been conducive to good decision making.

Morell was surprisingly late to diagnose Parkinson's disease (in those days referred to as paralysis agitans), or at least to document it, but did so three weeks before Hitler's suicide. In early 1945 Morell at long last diagnosed Parkinson's disease and indicated it in Hitler's medical chart. It should be noted that these

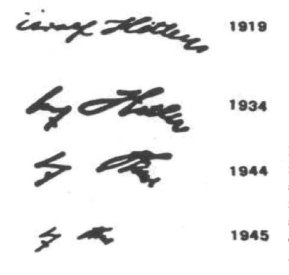

1919

1934

1944    Hitler's signature dete-
        riorated over the years,
        showing the progressive
        micrographia of Parkin-
        son's disease. (Reprint-
1945    ed with permission of
        Abraham Lieberman)

clinical features had already been observed by many of Hitler's nonmedical staff.

From my research I learned another characteristic finding of Parkinson's disease that Hitler displayed, micrographia (literally "small writing"), was disregarded or overlooked by Morell. Comparison of Hitler's signature from earlier in his life to that of the mid-1940s reveals dramatic changes. His signature in his later years showed the initial letter in the word written normally, or somewhat smaller than normal, followed by a severe tapering off in size and legibility of the remaining letters. His signature progressively worsened and typifies the micrographia of Parkinson's disease. Toward the end of his life his signature became so small and so cramped that it was illegible.

A 1945 newsreel by Swedish media escaped German censorship and represents conclusive evidence for Hitler's Parkinson's disease. In the clip Hitler demonstrates a coarse, slow, resting tremor of his left hand, diminished facial expression, and stooped posture and shuffling steps—all unmistakable and diagnostic features of Parkinson's disease.

Treatment of Parkinson's disease in the 1940s was severely limited. Curiously, Morell had for years treated Hitler's chronic gastrointestinal bloating and flatulence (most likely irritable bowel syndrome) with Dr. Koester's Anti-Gas Pills. This medicine inadvertently may have helped Hitler's hand tremor, as it contained a belladonna agent that would reduce Parkinson's tremor. Belladonna-like agents were the mainstay of treatment for Parkinson's disease before the advent of L-dopa treatment in 1968. For only the last two weeks of Hitler's life, Morell prescribed Homberg 680, a belladonna-like medicine, used at the time only to treat Parkinson's disease, along with subcutaneous injections of Harmin, also a belladonna-like medicine. In typical Morell fashion, if one medicine was good, three (including Dr. Koester's Anti-Gas Pills) must be even better.

**Behavioral Observations**

The motor features of Parkinson's disease have been well known since James Parkinson's original description in 1817, but its neurobehavioral effects received attention only during the past twenty-five years. In 1996 Vicki Soukup and Russell Adams determined the most consistently found cognitive impairment with Parkinson's disease was difficulty with concept formation, sequence planning, shifting and maintaining sets, and temporal ordering. In other words, people with longer-standing Parkinson's disease have difficulty shifting from one thought to another and in forming new ideas. In neuropsychological terms, this is a disorder of executive function and in neurological terms, a frontal lobe syndrome.

The behavioral syndrome of long-term Parkinson's disease differs from the better-known Alzheimer's disease in that the latter has a wider array of cognitive symptoms and is readily apparent to casual observers. The milder frontal lobe dysfunction in advanced Parkinson's disease may even escape the notice of family and close friends but still give rise to debilitating cognitive abnormalities.

David Irving's book, *The Secret Diaries of Hitler's Doctor*, provided additional insight based on interrogations of high Nazi officials into Hitler's impaired movements and behavior. Professor Karl von Eichen, who treated Hitler, revealed in his interrogation the following: "His [Hitler's] movements and reactions, both physical and mental, had become slower and he now trembled frequently."

From interacting with many hundreds of people with Parkinson's tremor, I saw firsthand the frustration and embarrassment suffered from hand tremor, the most visible and recognizable sign of the disorder. Some of my patients would place the tremulous hand in a pocket, hide it behind his or her back, or even sit on it. For someone as personally modest as Hitler was (he even refused to undress in front of Doctor Morell), this obvious sign of Parkinson's disease must have proved especially annoying, frustrating, and embarrassing. The perceived social stigma attached to tremor created his need to hide it and I believe must have proved upsetting for him.

Ear, nose, and throat doctor Erwin Giesing recalled how Hitler's hand shook so badly that he had to put it down on the desk and wait awhile before dashing off his signature in one scratchy flourish. Since Hitler was right-handed, this observation by Giesing confirms his disease had progressed to both sides of his body.

I imagine Adolf Hitler must have felt enfeebled by his overall muscular rigidity and slowness to initiate and carry out movements. For a man always in a hurry such as Hitler, the exasperation resulting from his stiff, slow, and tremulous movements must have at times proved overwhelming. Given that Hitler was constitutionally armed by rage, this additional burden likely worsened his outbursts of extreme anger.

Cognitive and memory problems also existed in Hitler. Colonel-General Heinz Guderian referred to Hitler's mental inflexibility by saying, "In February 1945, Hitler seemed absent-minded and unable to concentrate. He was exhausted and could barely move around. He still sensed the essence of contradictory reports, but had lost his mental flexibility and imagination."

Albert Speer, in his foreword to Leonard and Renate Heston's book *Adolf Hitler: A Medical Descent*, also described these changes. Extractions from Speer's 1953 notes characterized Hitler in 1938 as having allowed his associates to take full responsibility for their assigned fields and that Hitler accepted their conclusions without further examination. Later in the war Hitler began to avoid discussions, making decisions based only on his own views. Hitler seemingly became besotted with his own opinions and impervious to the opinions of others.

From the summer of 1942 onward, it struck Speer how rigid Hitler had become in his thinking. He described Hitler's mind as moving along an "unalterable track." Speer described Hitler as clearly having lost the mental agility of his earlier days. He lacked the capacity for thinking through large-scale conceptualizations, instead focusing on more trivial matters that should have been delegated to his, by then, frustrated generals. Speer described Hitler at this stage of his life as showing a "dull obstinacy."

These observations suggest the typical cognitive impairment now known to exist with chronic Parkinson's disease. At a time when Hitler was planning or executing troop deployments, the pathology of his Parkinson's disease was staging its own march through his undefended brain. The disease moved relentlessly through Hitler's brain stem and, later by way of subcortical pathways, outflanked his frontal lobes. The behavioral changes of Parkinson's disease in combination with Hitler's lifelong stubborn and paranoid personality, perhaps aggravated by amphetamine usage, resulted in impairment of his once crisp decision making. This deterioration in his mental abilities led to serious delays in his issuing orders and likely contributed to his egregious tactical errors.

**Impact of Hitler's Parkinson's Disease on the Battle of Normandy**
I propose loss of Hitler's mental flexibility and his inability to handle contradictory reports contributed to the outcome of the Battle of Normandy.

At 6:30 in the morning on June 6, 1944, Allied troops stormed the beaches of Normandy. The shaken German defenders, after gazing out on the massive Allied armada, immediately called for reinforcements, anticipating the release of the six Panzer units and the Fifteenth Army reserves from the Pas de Calais. The request was slow to reach Hitler, who tended to sleep late. Hitler may have suffered a sleep disorder seen with Parkinson's disease that consists of insomnia, slowness to arouse, and daytime sleepiness.

Hitler's well-known tendency to fly into rages may also have proved fortuitous for the Allies. Despite alarming reports streaming in from Normandy, Hitler's aides were slow to awaken him, apparently for fear of becoming targets of his fury. When Hitler finally awoke around midday and learned of the requests to release the armored Panzers and other reserves, he quickly denied them. Hitler believed the real invasion would come at the Pas de Calais and that the Normandy incursion was only an Allied tactical feint.

Allied deceptions designed to thin the German ranks at Normandy had fostered Hitler's misbelief as to the site of the invasion. On the second day of the Battle of Normandy, the Allies moved to solidify their shaky beachheads. While the German forces mounted a counterattack, the Fifteenth Army reserves and the six available Panzer divisions played no part in it. This limited German counterattack failed. Hitler continued to cling to his misbelief as tenaciously as the bark to a German oak tree.

Adolf Hitler was fifty-five years old, had suffered from Parkinson's disease for more than ten years, and proved unable to assimilate the overwhelming evidence that the major Allied attack was aimed at Normandy, not Calais. Within this emotional caldera of conflicting reports and under the usual fog of war, I believe Hitler felt overwhelmed. Due to his behavioral impairment from Parkinson's disease, he was slow to abandon his previous belief that the invasion site was Calais. He was also slow because of his lifelong stubbornness and inability to admit his own mistakes. His mind-set likely led to a slow, stubborn, and burning rage that required two long days to resolve, and two especially fortunate days for the Allies to solidify their tenuous beachheads.

Hitler had the final say as to the disposition of German divisions. He ignored the sensible demands of Field Marshal Rundstedt, the German commander in chief of the western theater of war. The reserve units were held back specifically by Hitler's order, failing to utilize the night of June 6–7 to move the German units forward. This delay allowed Allied bombers to inflict heavy losses on Axis troops and equipment even before encountering Allied ground forces.

On June 8, two full days after the invasion, Hitler reluctantly released the full German reserves. The Allies had by then dug in, off-loaded armor and additional combat and logistical troops, and were able to repel the German counterattack.

The presence of the Western Front at Normandy meant Germany then had two fronts to defend, stretching its military beyond its capabilities. The German loss at the Battle of Normandy likely determined the outcome of World War II.

Winston Churchill in *The Second World War: Triumph and Tragedy* attributed Hitler's slowness to respond to the Normandy invasion solely to the carefully orchestrated Allied deceptions. Churchill famously said that in wartime the truth was so precious as to have to be surrounded by a bodyguard of lies. No doubt Allied intelligence misinformation proved critical, but I doubt it entirely explains the German military delay.

In addition to intelligence deceptions, I believe Hitler's dithering resulted from his mental inflexibility, difficulty in shifting his thoughts, and diminished executive function due to Parkinson's disease. Hitler's mental inflexibility, blended with his natural intransigence and rage, created a perfect mental storm.

Hitler's failure to follow the advice of his top military commanders continued throughout the remainder of World War II. Hitler threw tantrums, dressed down associates, and replaced high-ranking officers for failing to follow his impractical orders. He did not accept information that ran counter to his prior fixed notions. Tragically, it led to further loss of life and property on all sides. Hitler steadfastly persisted with the war despite

Germany's near-hopeless situation that resulted from the degradation of its troop strength, armaments industries, and fuel-storage capacity.

I believe Hitler's rages increased the longer he had Parkinson's disease. Stifled by his Parkinson's disease and his lifelong temperament, Hitler proved incapable of effectively performing his duties as overall commander of the German armed forces. He made progressively poorer choices, relegating Germany to further needless destruction.

On June 20, 1944, Colonel von Stauffenberg and other conspirators made an unsuccessful attempt to assassinate Hitler. This grew from their frustration over Hitler's failure to act in a rational military fashion. At a briefing, Stauffenberg placed a bomb within a briefcase beneath a sturdy oak conference table. When it exploded, it drove splinters into Hitler's legs, singed his hair, punctured his eardrums, and tattered his clothing, but the desperate act failed to kill him. The coup d'état leaders had hoped to form a German government acceptable to the western Allies and prevent the Soviets from overrunning their homeland. Hitler's inability to accept the reality of imminent defeat, despite overwhelming evidence for it and the necessity to do so, would doom Germany to total defeat and destruction.

**Final Thoughts**

Parkinson's disease did not give rise to Hitler's virulent anti-Semitism, megalomania, and brutality—all personality characteristics formed well before his neurological disorder. Hitler was never demented, as might be seen with Alzheimer's disease, but exhibited a mild frontal lobe syndrome. This behavioral alteration affected Hitler's executive functions and reduced his ability to conduct effective warfare; however, it would not have influenced his ability to make ethical decisions. In brief, I believe Hitler was culpable for his horrible deeds.

This second front at Normandy proved a death knell for the Third Reich. When it fell the following year, the Third Reich that Hitler had boasted would last a thousand years had barely lasted for ten.

# Chapter 14
# ANGELS ON THE CEILING

*The mind is its own place, and in itself*

*Can make a heaven of Hell, a hell of Heaven*

—John Milton

Emerging from the fog, vague spirits slowly took shape only then to fade out and become indistinct. Sarah blinked her disbelieving eyes. The tiny figures distorted and transformed, taking on frightening features. Sarah's body tensed. Dread flowed through her thin body like an electrical current.

*What are they? Why are they hovering like vultures? I'm not dead yet, am I?*

Sarah Simpson, an independent-minded seventy-seven-year-old retired science teacher, lay in her recently acquired hospital bed, a place where she fully expected to die. A portable commode, suction machine, intravenous pole, oxygen tank, and lift chair surrounded her like annoying, overly solicitous servants. Her shrinking world had been reduced to four whitewashed walls and a ceiling full of ugly pipes in the basement of her old Victorian home. That particular rainy day in March was no different from previous months except for the shocking arrival of her morphing little ceiling-dwellers.

Sarah knew she was dying. How could she not? Her oncologist had explained her bleak chances for surviving her cancer. Still, in her heart Sarah imagined somehow she would beat the odds and once again tend her prizewinning rose garden and resume her regular bridge parties.

While Sarah's basement had proved dank and lonely beyond her expectations, she felt home hospice vastly preferable to her moving to a nursing home. Too many of Sarah's acquaintances had suffered horrible indignities in what she considered to be wretched and impersonal facilities. She would have none of it. If her basement was the only space large enough in her home to accommodate all the home medical equipment, then the basement it was.

On top of facing down cancer, she also coped with Parkinson's disease. This double health hex made her feel particularly unlucky. Her Parkinson's disease impaired her ability to move, while the cancer drained her limited energy. With her wry wit, she envisioned that if hit by a sudden rush of adrenaline, she would have to fight, as she could not summon the energy to take flight.

*There they are again. How hideous they are. What do they want with me?*

Sarah's emotional state verged on panic, witnessing the recrudescence of gnarly, bizarre creatures with huge black eyes that stared down at her from the ceiling. She jerked her head from side to side, trying to comprehend this assault that grew from one moment to the next. Anguished and troubled, Sarah felt vulnerable—unable to fight and unable to flee. Fear slaked her diminished stores of fortitude. She observed the strange nonhuman spirits deploy outward from the ceiling's dark corners, as if in formation. They spread like scurrying cockroaches across the ceiling, their initial ranks reaching the higher aspects of the basement's walls. There they halted, as if awaiting final orders from some unseen malevolent arch demon.

*Maybe I am dead and this is hell. That's it. I died in the night and landed in hell.*

It was then that a strangely familiar earthly noise interrupted her fearful ruminations. Heavy clumping sounds and the creaking of old stairs directed her attention toward the nearby stairway. A moment later from the darkened stairwell Jerry Brothers's shadowed, angular frame appeared. He strolled nonchalantly across the floor. His footsteps clicked on the polished gray concrete floor. Jerry, he told me later, circumnavigated the lift chair and avoided the oxygen line in order to approach Sarah's bedside.

"How're you doing today, Sarah?" Jerry said in his calm, rich baritone that contrasted with Sarah's higher-pitched, tinny voice that betrayed her attempt to maintain her composure.

"Gosh, Jerry, am I glad to see you," she gushed. "Thought I'd died and gone to hell. I was obviously wrong. No way you'd be in hell!"

Brothers laughed heartily. "Well, if I end up there, I'll at least see a bunch of my old friends."

Brothers had gained both knowledge and increased understanding since his early days in the ministry. His work at hospice had taught him both the frailty of the human condition and that a single theological approach did not address all the challenges his work presented. He had become expert in identifying character strengths in his dying patients. Much like a skilled bricklayer he had learned to construct their individual attributes into high ego-protecting walls to defend against the universal fear of dying.

When Jerry related this story to me, he said Sarah represented just such a challenge for him. She had attended church regularly and professed to be a believer in Christ. Nevertheless, Jerry had been challenged to connect her amorphous spiritual beliefs into a sturdy bulwark against her mushrooming fears. He knew of Sarah's adamancy against entering a nursing home, causing her relocation to the basement to accommodate the bulky medical equipment.

"Jerry, awful things just happened." Sarah's words spewed forth with brief, little sobs and sniffling that made her speech only partially intelligible.

"Now, now, Sarah. Tell me all about it. What's bothering you? I can be a good listener." Jerry's calming presence moved in closer to Sarah.

After a few moments she managed to blurt out, "I'm so scared of dying. I don't know what to expect. It could be terrible." She then broke into unrestrained sobbing, her thin chest heaving uncontrollably.

Jerry sat down in a poorly padded wooden chair and edged it closer to the bedside. He took her pale, wrinkled old hand within his warm hand and curled his elongated fingers around it. Jerry's clean-shaven, kindly face projected concern and love.

"Let's talk about it," he said, his other hand moving to loosen his stiff white collar. "We must recall that death is a fisherman, and we are the fishes. And you know who, of course, the real fisherman is." Jerry, he reported later, sensed her vulnerability and knew his help was needed like never before.

Understanding the significance of hallucinations for patients' lives remains a puzzle, but one worthy of further consideration. In my career, treating thousands of patients with Parkinson's disease, I encountered many who experienced vivid visual hallucinations. While for some their illusions were demonic and fear inspiring, for others, and more frequently, they consisted of angelic figures or quiet, observing sentinels. My patients sometimes interpreted the visitors as their "guardian angels."

Robert Roland, a sixty-three-year-old preacher, described to me two angels who intermittently would appear in his peripheral vision. He identified them as female, because they wore lovely, streaming white gowns. Their faces, however, remained for him indistinct. Robert referred to his visitors as "Goodness" and "Mercy" and he felt reassured and comforted by their presence. He believed "Goodness" provided him with unvarying kindness while "Mercy" supplied him with the compassion and forgiveness that as a Christian he sought.

This clergyman also related how his legs at times would not move and how "Goodness" and "Mercy" would intervene. Such immobility in advanced Parkinson's disease is referred to as freezing. A particularly inopportune freezing episode occurred one night when Robert was attending a meeting for Cowboys for Christ. He suddenly became unable to walk, as if his feet had been glued to the floor.

Robert saw "Goodness" and "Mercy" out of the corner of his eye, their bearings and presence suggesting to Robert their rising concern over his predicament. The cowboys in attendance noticed as well and began to debate how best to assist Robert. They became inspired to pray for Robert and to anoint his balky legs with the available cooking oil. Following the prayers and the anointing, Robert's legs again began to move normally. Robert believed his angels had miraculously effected the cowboys' healing actions.

Margie Freeman, a sixty-eight-year-old woman with Parkinson's disease, had always had an artistic bent, but she had not taken up painting until after developing her neurological disorder. The adoption of this creative endeavor was heroic, given the progressive impairment of her fine motor control. Nevertheless, she persisted despite her challenges and with the assistance of her guardian angel.

Margie described that while painting, she would see her guardian angel appear in the form of a little girl. The interest shown by the child encouraged Margie to overcome her impaired hands and to create lovely paintings.

On one occasion, as she sat sipping her afternoon tea, Margie became unaware that her teacup was precariously tilted and about to spill into her lap. The little girl glided silently forward and gently righted Margie's skewed teacup. Margie recognized that her sense of balance for her teacup had deteriorated and her guardian angel helped prevent her spilling her tea.

Three or four nicely dressed women would also visit Margie from time to time. These phantasms were extremely attractive. The ladies would sit sedately on her couch or in chairs near Margie. The elegant ladies, Margie said, would observe her unobtrusively and act attentively toward her. If Margie looked directly at them, or if Margie's husband happened to enter the room, the ladies would instantly dissipate like puffs of smoke in the wind. The visitors did not alarm Margie; on the contrary, they made her feel more self-confident.

Linda Mayfield, a seventy-two-year-old rancher from a dusty tumbleweed-rich, West Texas town, likewise experienced visual hallucinations with her Parkinson's disease. She also possessed an ineffable sense of humor and love of the comedic. Linda described a blond-haired girl who would climb onto the piano bench beside her. The girl had an uncanny resemblance to Linda at that early age and would observe her playing the piano. Linda believed the blond-haired girl was her guardian angel. Linda's angel provided comfort, encouragement, and much-needed company, but the little girl never spoke a word.

Linda described an unusual episode during her scheduled colonoscopy. Before receiving any preoperative medicine that might explain her unusual experience, she sensed the gurney on which she was lying begin to move erratically. Those in attendance tried to reassure her that the gurney was entirely stationary. Linda remained unconvinced, as she knew what she felt. She saw an animated man in a white coat running away in the opposite direction and down the hallway. She remained convinced that he had caused the sensation of movement. The episode provided Linda a sense of joviality due to her perception of orneriness by her white-coated guardian angel. The phantasm provided the comedic relief that she, with her well-developed sense of humor, needed to mitigate her anxiety about the colonoscopy.

How should we think about such episodes and the intercession of hallucinated guardian angels? From a descriptive point of view, these "angels" were faceless, usually benevolent, but at times teasing. They provided protection, assurance, or distraction. The silent guardians came in many shapes and sizes. Most merely observed the activities of the person but at times interceded, if the situation demanded it. They disappeared if gazed upon too directly or vanished from sight if someone else entered the scene. Attempts to touch them resulted in their instantaneous disappearance.

Most persons with Parkinson's disease with visual hallucinations accept their guests with little concern or fuss. They realize the hallucinations are not real and may take pleasure in them and exert a degree of control over them. When the lighting is poor or when consciousness is impaired, as with sleepiness or delirium, the chances for hallucinations increase. This limited control and the degree of pleasure derived suggest hallucinations may in part reside within the patients' control.

The medical literature provides little information regarding the nature of the nonthreatening hallucinations seen with Parkinson's disease. The medicines used to treat the disease are thought to be the principal cause of the visions. Hallucinations are seen most commonly with advanced disease and especially in older patients or with advanced disease where a degree of cognitive impairment exists. The ongoing bombardment of the receptors in the brain affected by Parkinson's disease may lead to hallucinations as well as to other side effects.

But a broader question presents itself: what possible purpose or mechanism could these angels serve in the lives of persons with Parkinson's disease?

Anthropology teaches that all cultures possess innate belief systems of a higher power. It is not too surprising that people suffering illness would hallucinate divine spirits consistent within their religious traditions.

The word *angel* derives from the Greek word for messenger. The ancient Greeks believed couriers existed to link mankind with their panoply of gods. More recently angels have been conceived as empowered for justice, guidance, and especially for personal protection.

Christianity is replete with references to angels. Within the New Testament, the angels gave messages to Joseph, Mary, and the shepherds. They ministered to Jesus during his temptation in the wilderness and visited him during his agony on the cross. Angels visited Christ's tomb and provided reassurance for those left aghast by their discovery of the empty tomb.

Angels were even more prevalent in the Old Testament. Many of us are familiar with Moses's encounter with God in the burning bush. The next two encounters in the Hebrew Bible involve the patriarch Jacob. The first consists of his battle with a figure that may have been an angel. The second occurs when Jacob climbs the unending ladder to heaven, which is held up by angels.

The Roman Catholic Church venerates archangels Michael, Gabriel, and Raphael by a feast each September 29. Catholics believe each person has his or her own guardian angel. The Eastern Orthodox Church mentions thousands of angels but provides names for only seven archangels.

Intriguingly, Raphael is described in Judaism as the archangel of healing. What a wonderfully appropriate derivation for a spirit who watches over people with health problems such as Parkinson's disease.

Islam has ten archangels, including Michael, who presented the Koran to Mohammad and induced him to read it. Angels in Islam are typically beautiful beings with wings. They are believed by the faithful to have been created before the existence of humans.

The Buddhist equivalent of an angel is a deva, also referred to as a celestial being. These angels are usually described as emanations of light or energy, but may be depicted in physical form. Devas are invisible to the human eye but can be detected by humans who have opened the *divyacaksus*, which is an extrasensory power through which one sees beings from other planes.

The angels of Christianity, Judaism, Islam, and Buddhism carry out various functions but all act as intermediaries between mankind and the divine. Of particular interest is that when angels appear to people in the various cultures, they do so in ways that are always culturally appropriate. Several weeks following the onset of Sarah's frightening hallucinations and after many visits and serious work by Chaplain Jerry, he returned for a follow-up visit.

"How ya doing, Sarah?" Jerry said after emerging from the stairwell and languidly approaching her cluttered bedside.

He scraped the old wooden chair across the concrete floor to her bed in order to hear her faint, strained, but more confident-sounding voice.

"Am doing better," Sarah said hoarsely. She paused for a moment to clear her throat. "The little people aren't changing anymore. They in fact have developed into the prettiest angels. They make me feel secure. Jerry, I no longer am afraid to die. I now realize the angels on the ceiling came to comfort me and keep me from harm. As you said, they will accompany me on the landing to the distant shore. No longer will I hurt or be troubled by this confounded tremor." Sarah directed her gaze toward her tremulous hands.

"You look to be at peace, Sarah. For this we can truly give thanks," the modest chaplain said. "Would you like for me to offer a prayer of thanks for your guardian angels?"

For Sarah the nonhuman spirits had stopped transforming themselves and had taken on the appearance of cherubic, red-cheeked angels and provided her with unconditional love and solace. The angels created in her a sense of calmness and certainty. Sarah had begun to welcome the extraordinary transition that lay ahead. Her hallucinated guardian angels had proved sufficiently powerful to rid Sarah of her greatest apprehension, the fear of dying.

Pastor Jerry's calming effect had laid a scaffold upon which Sarah's frightening hallucinations transformed into her idyllic guardian angels. He had, through his counsel, restructured the hallucinations from ominous to protective.

Jerry told me later that not long after his last visit, Sarah's health further deteriorated, and she died peacefully in the underground room of her home.

No doubt her guardian angels watched over Sarah during her final changeover from her living state to that which lay beyond. It was as Pastor Jerry had said: "Death is a door and not one we should fear passing through."

*Chapter 15*

# SAIL AWAY

*Hope, the patent medicine for disease, disaster, sin.*

—Wallace Rice

*I have been sustained throughout my life by three saving graces—my family, my friends, and a faith in the power of resilience and hope. These graces have carried me through difficult times and they have brought more joy to the good times than I ever could have imagined.*

—Elizabeth Edwards

The ship's horn boomed expectantly. The band played "Happy Days Are Here Again." Champagne glasses clinked, and peels of laughter crested and faded. Milling dockside relatives waved handkerchiefs. Then the ship's horn again blasted, increasing further our near-frenzied anticipation. Gray plumes began to billow from the huge smokestacks. It was just then that I felt it—a faint shuddering that pulsed the deck beneath my feet.

*Have the ship's engines really started or have the tremors of our Parkinson's party suddenly synchronized?*

It would be a never-to-be-forgotten cruise, but mostly for all the wrong reasons. I served as physician for a tottery band of intrepid travelers, a group that had stubbornly but bravely refused to cave in to their shared malady. It was February 2001;

we were aboard the *Gigantus*, the pride of the Mauritanian line (come to think of it, the *only* ship of the line still afloat). With the ship docked at the port of Fort Lauderdale, the crew scrambled about in expectation of sailing.

My planned but unannounced retirement was still six months away. Vicki, my fearless nurse practitioner, had once again connived me into serving as neurologist and educator for this indomitable group. As we stood on the top deck of the *Gigantus*, I reviewed our trembling charges. I felt shadowed by a metaphysical dread, resulting from a doubling in the number of Parkinson's disease patients compared to earlier cruises. News of the success of the prior sailings had spread like a contagion among national Parkinson's disease support groups, which contributed to our burgeoning numbers. I recalled the prior cruises had been largely without incident, providing me a modicum of reassurance. Their physicians had certified our travelers healthy enough for a cruise, but as I was to learn, these medical screenings may have been more procedural than precise.

Shuttling among our group, Vicki passed flutes of bubbly champagne. In her role as self-appointed pharmacist, Vicki also provided a chaser of antinausea patches. I was surprised that Melanie, our clinic nurse, was among Vicki's grateful recipients of a patch. Melanie hurriedly slapped the antimotion patch behind her right ear. I observed she already wore that telltale pallid, lemon-sucking facial expression of seasickness.

*And we've yet to depart the dock!*

My gaze fell on a button the size of a basketball that screamed in bold letters *Bush v. Gore — A Travesty*, pinned proudly to Vicki's jacket. When I tore my eyes away, I noticed Vicki had developed a perplexed look on her freckled face, her arm outstretched and frozen before a tiny, curled-over lady in a wheelchair. Vicki had proffered a glass of champagne that just then hung mid-air, Vicki's downcast gaze having locked onto a feeding tube that snaked from under the woman's blouse.

My eyes studied the wheelchair-bound lady located fifteen feet or so from me. I later was to learn that her name was Mary

and that she hailed from Minneapolis. Mary appeared frightful-
ly frail, but I felt encouraged by the presence of her attendant.
In addition to Mary's feeding tube, I also observed that she had
a tracheotomy and a catheter attached to a leg urine bag.

*How ever did she pass the medical screening?*

Mary discretely declined the champagne, avoiding further
embarrassment for Vicki. I chuckled, visualizing Vicki fum-
bling to administer champagne via the feeding tube—an act I
never doubted Vicki would have attempted.

With Vicki's twangy speech bubbling as much as the champagne, she scurried off in search of thirsty Parkinson's disease
travelers and still more ears to patch.

The following morning our group gathered for our initial educational session. Vicki and I were to be the speakers. I would
cover soon-to-be-released medicines for Parkinson's disease,
and Vicki would present the timely topic of dietary impact on
Parkinson's disease control. Vicki and I had a few minutes to
consider our program before our slow-moving traveling companions assembled in the ship's lounge.

"What's with the button?" I asked Vicki. Her message button
that day read "Save Nauru." Her myriad causes and buttons
had frequently prompted me to ask for additional explanation.
As I awaited her response, I felt the ship sway beneath my feet.

Vicki swished her curly red hair from side to side, as her
green eyes stared intently at me with an impatient what's-with-
you look. "Tiny Nauru's an island in the South Pacific, threatened by the greenhouse effect," she replied in the practiced
manner of an accomplished propagandist.

Vicki spritzed her words, and her explanation left me baffled. "What do greenhouses have to do with a Pacific island?"
I persisted.

"Global warming, melting ice caps, rising oceans, just a matter of time until poor Nauru disappears under the waves just
like Atlantis. Boss, you need to get out more. I feel responsible
for letting you and other people know what will happen, and,
well, I am kind of . . .prophetic."

*Prophetic, huh.*

"Gotcha," I said, nodding my head but truthfully not fully understanding. Members of our party continued to shuffle and shake into the lounge. I saw Bill Nelson, my patient of several years, heading down the aisle in our direction.

"How are you dealing with the movement of the ship?" I asked Bill, who was eyeing an empty seat in the front row.

"Well, now y'all know how we with Parkinson's feel," he quipped. "Not much different from every day on land. I've been known to stagger from pillar to post back home in table-flat Amarillo."

I saw Melanie clutching chair backs as she crept slowly down the aisle, seemingly having as much difficulty negotiating the ship's motion as were the patients. She plopped heavily into a deep red, thickly cushioned chair, wearing a spacey look and a big grin on her face.

*Well, she looks happy.*

Soon the group gathered and I gave my talk. My presentation went well. The FDA would soon release several medicines for treatment of Parkinson's disease, sparking interest among our consumers of vast quantities of pills, always on the lookout for promising new therapies.

Then Vicki took center stage. Vicki's talk focused on how excess protein in the diet counteracted the beneficial effect of L-dopa, resulting in worsening control of Parkinson's disease. Most of the guests on the cruise took some variety of L-dopa, the principal treatment for Parkinson's disease, so I knew her message was timely and important. She explained how the breakdown of protein prevented the normal transport of L-dopa to the brain where it was vitally needed to facilitate movement. She concluded her talk by saying that changes in diet such as increased intake (as may occur on a cruise, for example) could lead to worsening Parkinson's disease symptoms.

Vicki was and to this day is an excellent and entertaining presenter, interjecting the right amount of humor along with solid medical information. On scanning the audience, however, I noticed a number of dubious expressions. Questions from the audience suggested resistance to Vicki's wise advice. I chimed in supporting Vicki's well-intentioned and factually correct admonitions.

Nevertheless, the audience appeared to tune out our message of dietary moderation. I remember thinking that even had George Washington, Winston Churchill, Albert Schweitzer, and Jesus Christ all appeared as a panel with that ascetic message, still the patients would likely have turned as deaf as the figures on Mount Rushmore. *Guess this cruise is their vacation and restraint is hard to sell.* I feared our patients could not and would not resist the lavish feasts served daily. The immediate stick-to-your-ribs gratification would inevitably bat away Vicki's recommended moderation. For someone without Parkinson's disease, indiscretion might mean an extra five pounds. I feared for those with Parkinson's disease, major dietary changes would mean jackhammer tremor, slothlike slowness, and suit-of-armor stiffness. In addition to increasing their own suffering, by ignoring her message, many of our Parkinson's disease travelers would create long hours of work for Vicki and me during the cruise.

Two days later Trudy, Vicki, Melanie, and I stood at the deck railing overlooking the helipad, rubbernecking at the unfolding drama below us. A medevac helicopter hovered, then touched down on our ship's bucking foredeck. The personnel loaded a man on a stretcher, and shortly after, the helicopter lifted off, bound for a hospital in Miami. I thought the whole process went remarkably smoothly, too smoothly really, as if the drill had been frequently practiced.

It was then I determined to make a courtesy call on the ship's doctor. It turned out Doctor Heinz Crenwelge, an affable German surgeon, was inordinately happy to meet me. He had spotted our slow movers and shakers and feared he would be asked to provide them care. He was quick to admit he knew nothing about Parkinson's disease. I assured him that I would manage their Parkinson-related complaints.

"I noticed the air evacuation yesterday. Went without a

hitch," I said, as I sat on a tiny metal stool in a cramped exam room in the infirmary.

"Not unusual air evacs to have," said Doctor Crenwelge with his thick German accent. "Bevore da helicopter, da coronary care unit vas constructed, da man diedt." Raising his right brow, Heinz shrugged his shoulders and seemed largely nonplussed.

"Wow," I said. "Hadn't thought about people dying during a vacation cruise."

Heinz made a flicking movement of his fingers. "Passengers about deaths, dey know nothing," he said. And with a slight smile to one side of his mouth he continued, "Conzider age ovf mein pazzengers, many in dheir sefenties or eighties, zometimes wone hundred, dey come heir onboard zick, dey get vorse, und almost efery cruise zome die."

Before I left the infirmary that day, Heinz invited Trudy and me to join him later in the ship's bar. This would become a regular event to join Heinz and his attractive blond nurse, Katrina, for drinks before dinner.

Several days later and well after midnight, Trudy and I were called from the dance floor by the alarming message that Mary from Minnesota had suffered some type of an emergency. I asked Trudy to retrieve my black bag from our cabin and quickly departed the lounge. I then raced down multiple floors on thickly carpeted blue stairs until I located her cramped stateroom. On entering, I noticed Mary lying frighteningly still, her skin ashen. She was not breathing. Her attendant cowered nearby, wringing her hands.

Almost immediately I spotted a problem when I tried to use the suction machine. "This doesn't have the right plug, and it's for alternating not direct current," I said irritably. I threw down the useless plug and quickly examined Mary for any signs of life. Trudy had arrived by then with my black bag. I could detect no heartbeat. I felt no pulses. Her pupils were unreactive to a flashlight.

"I discovered that first day on ship," the attendant said sheepishly.

"Did you contact the ship's staff for a step-down converter and a different plug?"

"No, didn't think of that."

My attempts at resuscitation proved futile and short lived. Lacking resuscitation equipment, oxygen, paddles, and suctioning capability, my efforts were insufficient and useless.

The suction machine brought from Minneapolis had been equipped with a plug for American outlets, not the three-pronged European outlets on the ship. It became clear that Mary had not been suctioned in days and had slowly drowned in her own secretions.

We staff members had not noticed Mary's failure to appear at our recent educational sessions; the lectures being optional, not everyone attended. I regretted not having realized the challenges and risks that such a large party of advanced Parkinson's disease patients entailed. I felt a distinct sense of loss over Mary's death.

I was lost in thought when I noticed that Madge, Mary's caregiver, was speaking to me. "We better call her family," she said. "But I just can't do it."

"Do you have her contact information?" I asked.

"Her daughter lives in the Twin Cities. I have her number somewhere."

An hour later I found myself on the bridge of the ship, standing behind a white-clad officer at the wheel. I held what looked like a large, primitive phone but in reality was a modern ship-to-shore telephone. I heard a strange rising and descending whooping sound that made the whole experience feel surreal.

*What can I say to someone with whom I have never established any rapport? "Sorry about the middle-of-the-night call, and oh, by the way, your mother just died."*

After almost three decades of medical practice, I had gained experience speaking with families about terminal diagnoses, horrific illnesses, vegetative states, and death. I did not doubt my ability to carry out this awkward task, but felt ill at ease not knowing the person with whom I was to speak and not knowing very much about the deceased herself.

The far-away phone in Minneapolis rang multiple times. Mary's daughter sleepily answered the phone after the fifth ring. "Hello," she slurred. She listened without interruption to my introduction and description of her mother's circumstances.

"I am so sorry to inform you that your mother passed away earlier tonight," I said as sympathetically as possible over the rising and falling whooping sound on the phone. There was a prolonged pause on the line. Had she collapsed or fallen back asleep? Had the connection been broken? I felt my mind becoming more restive still.

"Suspected she wouldn't make it," was the daughter's eventual laconic reply. She suddenly sounded fully awake.

*Didn't think she would make it. What? Then why put her on a cruise ship and scare the hell out of me? She didn't need a Caribbean cruise—she needed an intensive care unit!*

"I am really not surprised, but my mother so wanted one final exploit. She wore us down, hired Madge on her own, and finagled a medical approval from her all-too-compliant doctor. She was always the determined one."

I felt myself intrigued by the tenacity of this sprite of a woman who had gone to such lengths to travel. "Tell me more about your mother. Unfortunately, I did not have a chance to get to know her very well," I said. Outside, the ship passed through a squall line with raindrops pounding against the glass windows of the bridge. This only contributed to the seeming unreality of the moment.

"She is, sorry, was, an original piece of work. On her seventieth birthday, she went skydiving. Can you believe it, jumping out of a perfectly good airplane with only a parachute and in her condition? Last year she rode a balky burro named James into the Grand Canyon. Another year she had herself strapped on a dogsled and mushed across Alaska. Never one to give in to her Parkinson's disease that's for sure. A real adrenaline junkie, just loved risky experiences, said it made her feel alive."

"Her determination sounds inspiring," I said.

"Mother leaned into risks. Said she would regret not trying

her adventures more than if something unfortunate was to happen."

"Wow, that's impressive. Thanks for sharing. I had no idea," I said. This back story from the daughter had in fact substantially altered my perception of Mary.

"No reason for you to know. People in Minneapolis heard about her exploits, though. Jim Klobuchar, a columnist for the *Minneapolis Star and Tribune,* wrote about her daredevil, never-give-in-to-illness lifestyle. Weird to have people approach me after that. Folks I barely knew told me how much they admired Mother's courage."

The conversation ended with our agreement to speak again about arrangements for handing over Mary's body. The daughter indicated she would ask her brother to fly down to the Caribbean and collect the body at a port yet to be determined.

Earlier, Doctor Crenwelge had arrived in Mary's cabin following the failed resuscitation and facilitated the middle-of-the-night call to Minneapolis.

"Heinz, what should we do with the body until the family picks it up?"

"In dis hot climate, is imposzible in a stateroom to keep," he said while making a gesture of pinching his nostrils. "Ve must put dis voman in a cool place."

"Have we a mortuary on board?"

With a detached demeanor, he replied, "Nein, ve vill put da boty on ize in da refricheraytor."

"You mean in the refrigerator with the leftover vegetables and desserts?" I exclaimed disbelievingly.

"Yah, dere iz lotz ovf room; it is a bick refricheraytor." At that point, I gulped audibly. After his solution, the buffets for me never looked quite so appetizing.

Our next scheduled stop was Martinique, a French island. This port prompted certain, shall we say, sensitive political considerations.

Heinz took me aside the following afternoon, physically separating me from my traveling companions. "Tohm, vhile in

Martinique, ve can't tell dem ovf da boty on da boot." Heinz said this in a conspiratorial voice and with a concerned look on his clean-shaven, square face.

"Why not?" I asked. My vision of a body bag in the food cooler was not at all pleasing.

"Da gofernment bureaucrats might hold da ship, vfor maybe a veek. Ve can't let vord slip aut or ve vill be baried in red tape. The next port avter—St. Thomas, American Virgin Islands— dhere ve can tranzfer da boty."

Spoiling vacations for several thousand vacationers, all of whom were oblivious to Mary's death, would undoubtedly have prompted a horrific outbreak of shipboard crankiness. I felt uneasy agreeing to this deception but finally determined to keep our, by then, cold little secret. Nevertheless, the following day, as we pulled into the port at Martinique, I was mindful of the body bootlegged deep within the ship's refrigerator.

The following day I accompanied half of our traveling group on a tour of that beautiful Caribbean island. Vicki went with the remainder for a day at a white sand beach. That day Vicki determined the division of labor by saying she wanted to seriously work on her suntan. I clucked to her that her outing would only likely prompt a fresh crop of freckles and sunburn.

Later that afternoon I saw Vicki in a skimpy flowered swimsuit running helter-skelter up the gangway. I knew from watching her churning legs that something must have gone seriously awry.

"Vicki, what's up?" I said, as I hurried toward the gangway to meet her.

"George Fisher, the PSP patient, drowned!" Vicki's green eyes flashed and her usually animated state had rocketed well into the stratosphere.

"You mean he's dead?"

"Not a chance, not with ole Vicki on the job. Got him to the beach, turned him upside down, and drained about five gallons of saltwater out of him."

George Fisher had a disorder more severe than Parkinson's

disease known as progressive supranuclear palsy (PSP). One difference from Parkinson's disease is that with PSP the neck becomes extremely stiff and usually assumes a flexed and immobile position. Seems George Fisher wanted to snorkel that morning (a sport he had never previously experienced), but an activity poorly tolerated when water is inhaled and an inability exists to lift the head from the water.

"How did you get George out of the water?"

"Remembered my lifesaving and drug him to the water's edge. Some nice French folks moved him a little farther onto the beach.

I thought her exploit was nothing short of amazing, especially given Vicki's diminutive size and George Fisher's heft.

"Where's he now?" I asked.

"Martinique EMS arrived, intubated him, and hauled him to their hospital," she said, as she bounced around in place.

Mrs. Fisher had accompanied him on the cruise, I recalled. *At least I won't have to make another difficult phone call to the mainland.*

"I need a drink, something really strong," Vicki said. "And, boss, I expect you to buy."

"I'll pay and for as much as you want," I said guiltily, knowing I had drawn the easier shore duty that day.

A few minutes later we entered one of the many bars on the ship. We noticed Heinz and Katrina at a table with empty places. They spotted us and beckoned us to join them. Trudy, Vicki, and I took our seats and exchanged pleasantries.

In short order, Vicki shared her drama from the day and began to drain one rum punch after another. She said that she had focused her attention on an elderly lady with PD who for the first time in her life had wanted to swim. What had concerned Vicki was that the lady had no idea how to swim or even float. While demonstrating an admirable adventuresome spirit, the distraction had unfortunately directed Vicki's attention away from George Fisher who by then, no doubt, was flailing face-down in the surf.

"Say, this ssstuff is gooood. This is what Melanie's been

drinking and pretty gooood too," said Vicki, her words slur-ring. "Melanie finds, if she's just a little bitty drunk, doesn't feel sooo seasick."

*So that's why Melanie has had that goofy smile on her face? Ex-plains why she's been staggering too. Had no idea Melanie suffered from motion sickness or had a fondness for rum punch.*

Given Mary's death and the near miss on George Fisher, talk at the table soon turned to similar matters aboard ship. Heinz had gone to sea years before and had experienced many unusu-al shipboard events. After several Grolsch beers, he began to share cases that had not gone well and some that had died and required burials at sea.

"No way, people still bury at sea?" I asked incredulously.

"Zsure do, efery so offen," Heinz said. "Ve vonce had an en-tire family come on da boot to bury dheir grandpa in da briny deep zee."

"Tell me you're kidding?" I said.

"Vish I vas," Heinz replied. "Ve had not buried anyvon re-cently, zo an hour before da ceremony, I vanted da body slide checkt. Ve loaded it wit dheir opa tucked inside hiz body bag. I hat doubt ivf de handle vfor da slide vorked. On da springh mechanism, I squirted zome oil and pulled to loozen da handle. Vhoops! Da zleide vorked fery gute, but bevore I could stop da body frohm going down da zleide, it vent into da oashen und splashed. Imagine da surprise I hat?"

"And all this was before the family had arrived or the cere-mony performed?" I asked.

"Bad situvation vor sure," Heinz said. "I wondered what to do wit no body unt a family vanting vfor a funeral. Dhen to me it came, I could fill a boty bag vit potatoes frohm de kitchen. Da family would know nothing. Zo, I took da bag und filled it wit potatoes und onions, und put it on da zleide."

Vicki, who was looking toasted at that point, Trudy, and I sat listening with rapt attention. "Well, what happened?" I asked.

"Vell, avter prayen und singen vfor long time wit da grieven family—dhose potatoes und onions got a gudt und proper buri-al, dey did. Ve made a nice funeral ve did, as gudt as you haf seen, complete with da ship's band played 'Amadzing Grace,' vich da family said vas dheir opa's favorite. Da family vas nefer viser und on da vay out, complimented how lofely de funeral vaz."

Regardless of nationality, physicians and nurses have their own weird sense of humor. I suppose its morbid tone stems from dealing with many sad situations and the need to reduce their levels of stress. In any event, the story struck those at the table as hilarious. We laughed till tears rolled down our cheeks, and the shared moment prompted another round of drinks.

By then the rum punches had caused Vicki to develop hiccups that began to punctuate Heinz's storytelling.

"On anoder occasion just as da body down the slide slid, we heard rumbling from da kitchen below."

"Hic."

"All da ship's staff recognized da noise: the kitchen its garbage purging. Sure nuf we droppedt dat body into the ocean right along with da garbage. Fortunately, da family didn't know, but da staff to keep straight faces hard to do."

"Hic." Vicki placed her tiny hand over her mouth and smiled guiltily.

"Tell dem about spreading da ashes, Heinz," Katrina urged, her expressive brown eyes filled with mirth.

A smile spread across Heinz's broad face, anticipating his retelling of the story. "One family arrifed wit da urn ovf Aunt Joyce's ashes at sea scatter. Several hat lovely stories about dheir Aunt Joyce who lovet to cruise. On da ship, you know, ve paint a lot. Salt air eats da paint. Da vhite paint on da back of da ship dat day vas still vet. Vhen da solemn moment came Aunt Joyce's ashes to scatter, a strong gust ov vind blow da ashes back against da vet paint. Dhose ashes against da hull dey stuck. Frohm den to now, Aunt Joyce vit us has been sailing. Kind of like a forefer fwee kruse, you might zay."

The humorous stories proved to be cathartics for our troubled minds. Heinz and Katrina had lightened our residual somber attitudes. I suppose this had been their intent all along.

When describing my memories of the cruise, I recognize that

no memory can be entirely accurate. Inevitably with memories, details are forgotten or exaggerated and influenced by the emotions they provoked. But in thinking back to that sailing in 2001, I distinctly recall several kernels of truth that took up residence deep within the chambers of my heart.

The principal heartfelt message was the courage displayed by our fellow travelers with Parkinson's disease. With rare exception, these gallant people did not complain, nor did they shy away from the educational and demanding shore excursions.

Molly, who was in her late twenties, had prominent twisting of her muscles, the so-called dystonic form characteristic of young-onset Parkinson's disease. The cruise offered her the opportunity to venture out with others with the same condition. And make the most of the trip she did!

She participated in every excursion, every onboard ship activity, and every seminar. She competed in shuffleboard and in the on-deck putting contests. I danced with her on the rolling deck one evening, her face aimed at the stars, radiating long-overdue pleasure.

While our Parkinson's group members did not always display resistance to the temptations in the restaurant, even when indiscretions brought about increased physical challenges, they showed determination and good humor.

Jonny Humphries became so slowed from his Parkinson's disease that he required a wheelchair for the tours, yet he refused to miss even a moment of the shore excursions. Gladys Barker became so stiff in her movements that she fumbled interminably to pull bills from her purse, but shop she did and transported enough gifts home to spike up the Caribbean economy.

As displayed by their presence on the cruise, this fearless band refused to give in to their infirmities. They indeed had reserved their places at a banquet of consequences.

No one exemplified this intrepidness more than Mary from Minneapolis. At a time when many with her level of problems would have occupied a bed in a nursing home, the undaunted Mary planned new adventures and challenges. As her daughter said with both pride and a tinge of regret, "We knew she needed the adventures but worried that she might not make it through alive. But it was her call, and she would never let her illness whip her. She was just like that, always had been."

The *Gigantus* docked at the final port on our cruise—San Juan, Puerto Rico. Trudy, Vicki, Melanie, and I stood near the top of the gangway, giving hugs to each of our slow-moving group and providing them with hand luggage or wheelchair assistance. The predictable breaks between their departures provided us a few moments to reminisce.

*The cruise flyers referred to me as an educator. Yet, I've learned more from our patients about personal courage and determination than I ever could have taught them. Makes me wonder, who were the real educators on the cruise?*

That day, Vicki wore a large button with green-and-red lettering on a white background, spelling the words "Ciao, y'all." I knew this Italian word, like the Hawaiian word *aloha*, carried multiple meanings and was often used as a greeting.

I felt pangs of hidden regret, stemming from my unannounced retirement that was known only to Trudy. I would miss the affirming and intimate interaction with people who had become friends and who had chosen to place their medical trust in me. I would miss those special professional caregivers and friends with whom I had worked, struggled, and sometimes cried.

Nevertheless, I felt the need for increased personal time and the opportunity to spend more time with my family. Just like these intrepid people with Parkinson's disease who refused to be defined or limited by their illness, I also craved an expanded life beyond my definition as a physician. I desired a phase in my life to pursue personal interests that had in recent years become increasingly difficult to tamp down.

I glanced at Vicki's button one more time. "Ciao, y'all." Her message showed Vicki's ready wit, to be sure, but that was not all. *Ciao* commonly meant hello but it also had a lesser-understood, nuanced meaning of good-bye or so long.

*Maybe Vicki really is prophetic.*

# AFTERWORD

The whirligig that was my professional life ended in 2001. Reaching this corner of my life allowed me to retire my black medical bag, begin new pursuits, and spend time reflecting on my forty years of practicing medicine. Nevertheless, memories of my patients' struggles, insights, and courage continued to haunt me; their voices, soft but plaintive, elbowing their way to the front of my mind. They demanded their stories be told. Those described herein have now either passed on or can no longer speak their narratives. I hope my telling does justice to the rich tapestry of their stories.

Time has moved on, prompting me to update the whereabouts of my mentors and colleagues. Doctor Bill Powell, the gentle and easygoing physician who introduced me to medicine, passed away in 2009. Regrettably, I lost track of him but suspect he proved successful and avant-garde in his later undertakings. Thank you, Doctor Powell, for your inspiration. Like the fate of many great teachers, you unknowingly set the course for my vocational journey.

Only two years following my fellowship on the US-USSR Health Exchange Program, Doctor A. R. Luria died in 1977 of heart disease. He had earlier barely survived the Stalinist purges and rabid anti-Semitism that had claimed the life of his closest colleague and friend, Lev Semionovich Vygotsky. Luria's death cut short his lifelong dream of providing a unified theory of psychology based on neuropsychological principles—an area he pursued during the final years of his life. His case studies of the two patients discussed in the acknowledgments to this book, one with phenomenal memory abilities and the other who suffered the tragic results of a traumatic brain wound, illustrate his blending of classical patient storytelling with experimental clinical approaches. He left behind exceptional work that provides an understanding of brain localization of higher cortical functions such as speech, spatial functions, memory and executive function, and the interaction of brain and its derivative, mind. Thank you, Alexander Romanovich.

My mentor in neurology, Doctor A. B. Baker, eventually stepped down as chairman of the Department of Neurology at the University of Minnesota. He had built an internationally renowned department that never felt quite the same without his steady hand on the tiller.

Regrettably in his later years, Doctor Baker succumbed to Alzheimer's disease. How ironic for a man with his neurological acumen to fall prey to a brain disorder. He, no doubt, possessed a hunch in the early stage of his illness of what stalked him. His intelligence and experience masked his disease from others for a longer period of time than possible for others less neurologically sophisticated. Always the master diagnostician, he eventually rendered his own, regrettably all-too-accurate diagnosis, assuming in his bigger-than-life persona both sides of the doctor-patient relationship.

Doctor A. B. Baker's impressive legacy consists of founding the world's largest neurological association—the American Academy of Neurology—training hundreds of neurologists, and contributing a trove of important research findings. I know physicians and the future of medicine will miss his commanding presence.

My colleague who is the basis for the character of Vicki Masters continues to provide compassionate care and insightful education for patients and their families. She continues to treat people with Parkinson's and Alzheimer's disease with her special sense of purpose and determination. She remains a close friend, visits periodically, and continues to needle me whenever I begin to take myself too seriously.

My own family members have matured during the time arc of the book. A young Katie may have learned more listening to my stories and hearing me practice lectures than I had realized at the time. She maintains her informal diagnostic skills, even today spotting people with Parkinson's disease while working in the Department of Continuing and Professional Education at Southern Methodist University.

Earlier in the chapter on Adolf Hitler I mentioned the television programs in which I speculated on the role his Parkinson's disease may have played on World War II. Admittedly I was proud at appearing in the shows and contributing my medical observations to history. During one weekend, we played the first video for the family to watch. I thought Katie, my daughter, would surely be impressed with her father's insightfulness or diagnostic acumen or at least that he was appearing on an international TV program. Instead she could only respond, "Dad, those glasses are *sooooo* old-fashioned!" How quickly our children burst our bubbles. (I did get new glasses shortly afterward.)

Andy became an attorney and for a while practiced medical malpractice defense (had he worked for the plaintiff side, I would have disowned him). I humor myself by thinking I influenced his initial focus in the law. He is now a partner in his own law firm. Neither Andy nor Katie wished to become physicians, witnessing all too closely its rigors. Medicine is not for everyone, although in my opinion the profession remains the best possible education to learn about life and people.

Trudy has continued to be a loyal, uncomplaining, loving, and independent wife. But fearing in retirement I might attempt to organize her activities and worrying about my being underfoot, she encouraged me to find replacement undertakings. Now this lifelong "city boy" owns a cattle ranch in the Hill Country of Texas, an activity that consumes time faster than a puppy can lap up spilled milk. On managing a cow/calf operation using cow dogs, I began as a blank slate. This created novel challenges that led to a broken arm, ruptured disc, torn ligaments, and bruised ego, but also provided a fun way to spend my time and a ready target for my fondness of living things.

Like many busy people, I found myself substituting activities in retirement to fill the available time. This included chairing the city/county health board, participating in medical missions to Mexico and Central American countries, and serving on the local hospital board. A particularly meaningful recognition came when I received a Lifetime Achievement Award from the Texas Neurological Society, a group with which I had a long and fulfilling relationship.

Following relocation from the Twin Cities, Dicey Dog, the incorrigible and overgrown Dalmatian, continued to provide my family with many belly laughs, as well as security for our Lubbock home. Regrettably, the dog's overprotectiveness of Katie prompted a second relocation for Dice to a Dalmatian breeding farm. As Trudy was fond of saying, "Dice went on to a *happier* life."

Not long after I completed my internship at Hennepin County General Hospital in 1973, the Old General was torn down. In its place rose a modern medical center with comfortable patient rooms and private offices for both staff doctors and house staff. With its new configuration, the unique and grand spirit of the Old General proved harder to sustain. Perhaps this resulted from physicians cubby-holed in their offices in contrast to the earlier crowded, collective experience. The Old General had something special about it, something intangible but truly wonderful. The spaces in which we performed our labors dictated how we did our work. The substandard physical conditions caused us not only to work together but also to pull together, enabling better solutions for the health-care challenges we faced.

Likewise, a spanking-new facility replaced the old Minneapolis Veterans Hospital. The VA system, once a model of inefficiency and the butt of jokes, later established the first nationwide electronic health records. No longer could a handful of veterans receive seasonal free room and board at different VA hospitals while serially undergoing evaluations for the *very same* medical condition.

A provision of the Patient Protection and Affordable Care Act of 2010 called for electronic health records throughout the entire country. The successful precedent from the Veterans Administration heralded this aim. The VA system has also become one of the leaders in the country in quality of care and patient safety. These two values have correctly become the guiding North Star for American medicine. In light of recent reports of long waiting times for patient care, timely access will now need to be addressed at some VA medical centers in a similar forward-looking fashion.

In reviewing these chapters, I am struck by my early naiveté and driven nature. This contrasts with later in my career when I found myself needing to ponder the richness of my patients' stories. The bedside and the area beside the exam table became for me something more than mere exam space. These small expanses became hallowed ground—ground that allowed me to delve into the core of my patients' lives and attempt to make a difference.

Patients taught me much about the human spirit. They educated me on how to listen, really listen. These patients through their bodily betrayals provided slivers of opportunity for insight and points of connection when I least expected them. Their stories about life-changing illnesses reveal much about the human condition, especially the sustaining power of love, faith, and hope.

The impact of love shines through their stories and demonstrates how very fortunate and rare it is to benefit from unconditional love. Too often what passes for love comes as a reward for worldly success. The aged, unattractive, but deeply bonded couple described earlier provides a different take on this and prompts our contemplation of the resilience of love and its importance for adding meaning to our lives.

Faith plays an important role in the health-care realm and

can augment both the effort of caregivers and perhaps even the outcomes of illnesses. Through the restructuring of a fearful patient's thoughts, a skilled chaplain was able to transform the fearful aspects of dying into a comforting transition to that which lay beyond. In recent years hospice services have embraced this restructuring approach and have broadened the scope of health care. Faith plays an important role not only in the lives of patients but also in the lives of health-care workers, as they struggle to understand and combat the ravages of disease.

Medicine has seen wonderful advances, but we must hope its practitioners will never forget the necessity of good communication among the health-care team and all that goes into the web of tangible and intangible interactions among doctors, patients, and other health-care professionals. The special relationship that exists between doctor and patient is like no other. It mixes trust, respect, hope, faith, and fidelity to what is best for the patient. The doctor-patient relationship is, after all, a one-on-one relationship but requires an entire team of cohesive members to ensure the highest-quality clinical outcomes.

If we allow ourselves to enter personally into these narratives, they inevitably draw attention to our own frailties and mortality, but they also demonstrate the hidden reservoirs of strength, courage, or in the instance of Adolf Hitler, abject venality that may reside within some people. Some of the stories demonstrate the wonderfully odd peculiarities that at times accompany brain disease. The out-of-kilter brain is capable of producing intriguing, insightful, and amusing actions. Such instances add fascination to neurology and highlight its similarity to sleuthing in other areas of human endeavor.

Over a professional lifetime I gained immense respect and awe for human life with all its complexities, humor, and heroism. This grew from improved understanding of patients, their caregivers, and their companions as they faced serious illnesses. Hopefully these stories will inspire further understanding of the need and power for physicians and laypeople to know and affirm the mysterious links between mind and body.

I acquired increasing respect, falling little short of idolatry, for the many "chosen ones"—family members who care for loved ones. Through selfless service, many family caregivers convinced me of the near-boundless capacity humans possess in caring for their loved ones. And as pointed out earlier, the loyal companion need not necessarily be human, but instead may have four paws and a wet nose.

I need to add a final clarifying word regarding one aspect of this book. As a senior medical student at Baylor College of Medicine, I received my first medical black bag. I felt as proud of the black bag as when Doctor Michael E. DeBakey, president of Baylor College of Medicine, handed me my medical diploma. My black bag provided a stamp of legitimacy and professionalism, even more so than did my white doctor's coat. It was a special symbol of the healing arts and, in contrast to white coats, was limited solely to physicians. Over the years, I continued to carry my exam instruments in my black bag.

This quaint custom of carrying a black medical bag has fallen from favor since my graduation from medical school. Perhaps black bags were thought unnecessary in the era of modern imaging and laboratory-intensive medicine due to the unfortunate de-emphasis of medical history taking and physical exam skills.

But for the practice of neurology, the black bag continues to serve an important function. The neurological examination still requires careful history taking and the use of instruments to perform the examination. Neurology provides a bridge between the more anachronistic but personalized focus on history taking, careful examination, long-term doctor-patient relationship, and the modern imaging and laboratory-intensive practice of medicine.

Admittedly, the black medical bag also became something of a signature for me. Many times I heard nurses or families exclaim, "We always know when you're on the floor [or in the clinic or wherever] when we see a black bag." To my knowledge when I took down my medical shingle, my black bag was the last one in use in Lubbock.

When I retired from medicine, my black bag traveled with

me to my ranch. There I placed my original ebony companion on my study shelf where today it peeks over my shoulder and resurrects fond memories. It is only fitting my black bag makes its appearance in many of these stories, as it represents to me much of what is good and eternal about the field of medicine.

At some point, most of us will face personal health challenges. I hope these medical vignettes will prompt more reasoned and comfortable consideration of how to face such challenges and will assist in maintaining personal dignity despite the inconvenience or threat of terminal illness. Let us be inspired by the grace, courage, and poise shown by many of those depicted within this volume. If this salutary effect occurs, then my effort in writing this book will not have been in vain.

# INDEX

# ABOUT THE AUTHOR

**Tom Hutton, MD,** is an internationally recognized clinical and research neurologist and educator. The past president of the Texas Neurological Society, Dr. Hutton served as professor and vice chairman of the Department of Medical and Surgical Neurology at the Texas Tech School of Medicine. He now lives on his cattle ranch near Fredericksburg, Texas.